INTO THE STORM

"*A powerful and moving book.*"

JOANNE SILBERNER

Former NPR national health correspondent

Collin Tong

— EDITOR —

"In the aftermath of his wife's devastating loss of memory, a struggle that ended with her death to Alzheimer's in 2011, Collin Tong's book reflects the importance of hearing the stories of other caregivers. Finding common ground in their struggles, *Into the Storm* wonderfully narrates how each summoned the courage to weather the impact of this frightening disease, thereby advancing our understanding of the caregiving process.»
> – *ROBERT C. JOHNSON*, Graduate School and Research,
> Gallaudet University, Washington, DC

"Albert Schweitzer spoke about 'the fellowship of those who bear the mark of pain.' Swept into this fellowship are persons with Alzheimer's disease, and also their caregivers. The enormous investment of care required of all who support and serve their stricken loved ones is described in these pages, beginning with Collin Tong's own story. Remarkable testimonies to the human spirit are evident, proving that pain is not the final word after all."
> – *DR. JOHN H. TOWNSEND*, Minister Emeritus,
> The First Baptist Church of Los Angeles

"Collin Tong has deftly accomplished what few do well—integrate his own personal experience with the stories of others who have struggled, and back that up with solid research—to present a cohesive and compassionate guide to caregiving for those struggling with Alzheimer's. This is a resource that will offer solace and strength to those who find themselves in the crucible of one of life's most difficult challenges—caring for a loved one who slips away in the long night of dementia. Collin gently offers guidance and hope as one who has walked that path."
> – *THE VERY REV. DR. STEVEN L. THOMASON*, Dean and Rector,
> Saint Mark's Episcopal Cathedral, Seattle, Washington

"*Into the Storm* reflects Collin Tong's journey as a caregiver and his dedication to connecting people in order to create an everlasting 'community of care' for those with Alzheimer's disease—and those who love someone living with it. Like the care experienced in a support group, *Into the Storm* powerfully depicts the lived experiences of caregivers and will be invaluable for families on that journey.
> – *PATRICIA HUNTER, MSW*, Washington State
> Long-Term Care Ombudsman

Acclaim for

INTO THE STORM

"When my father had Alzheimer's, I read every book I could find. I wish *Ir* *the Storm* had been available. The two dozen personal stories are sometim painful, sometimes joyful—but always helpful. You'll learn that you're r alone and, as unbelievable as it might sound, that there can be gifts throu the pain. A powerful and moving book."

– *JOANNE SILBERNER*, Former NPR national health correspond

"As this collection so richly documents, when a parent or life-partner is flicted with Alzheimer's, the full panoply of negative thoughts can afflict – from a sense of unfairness of the fates, to a feeling of being alone; to a p found experience of loss – and on…and on. Leo Tolstoy once famously wr that each family's troubles are its own – but to absorb the messages in t volume is to understand that Tolstoy's opening lines of *Anna Karenina* only partly true – that instead the common thread that builds our humai comes from actively engaging the support of others. And that comes if when we seek it."

– *TROY DUSTER*, Chancellor's Professor, Earl Wai
Institute of Law and Social Po
University of California, Berk

"Those of us who have lived through the Alzheimer's journey with a loved know how uncertain and all-consuming it can be. The personal stories ge ously shared by others were the saving grace for our family as we suppo my father on his own journey. This amazing collection is a gift to anyone ing for a loved one with Alzheimer's, or for those interested in enriching deepening their understanding of this disease."

– *DEBORAH SWETS*, Vice President of Member:
Washington State Hospital Associa

"For the increasing number of families experiencing Alzheimer's ease, these stories are a gift. Olivia Ames Hoblitzelle writes about the 'gra diminishment,' adding her voice to these other courageous authors who hope that we can live lovingly through the diminishment. *Into the Storm* essential book. "

– *GERRI HAYNES*, Past President, Washington Physicians for S
Responsibility and former Director of Palliative Nui
Evergreen Hospital Medical Center, Kirkland, Washir

"Wisdom resides in these stories, first-hand experiences that illuminate the path, helping the reader to calibrate and recalibrate, catch one's breath, and remember the vital importance of self-compassion. Kudos to Collin Tong and his extraordinary collaborators for the wealth of authentic guidance, road maps, and rest stops along this journey, conveyed in *Into the Storm*."

– *ROGER ROFFMAN*, Professor Emeritus of Social Work,
University of Washington

"We go into the storm, but not alone. With this book you will find new companions for the journey. Because we live out of stories, this work provides rich resources, not only for sustaining us but also to open us to the gift of new life in the face of loss."

– *REV. DR. ROBERT B. WALLACE,* Senior Pastor,
First Baptist Church of Claremont, Claremont, California

Collin Tong

INTO THE STORM

COLLIN TONG is a correspondent for *Crosscut News* and *University Outlook* magazine. He is also a Seattle-based stringer for *The New York Times*. He served as senior director for communications at Washington State University, guest lecturer at the Edward R. Murrow College of Communication at WSU, and public affairs director for the Alliance for Education. A former Michele Clark Fellow at the Robert C. Maynard Institute for Journalism Education, Tong was named the 2010 Volunteer of the Year by the Western and Central Washington State Chapter of the Alzheimer's Association and received the Katryna Gould Award for consumer advocacy by the National Adult Day Services Association. The University of Redlands conferred its Distinguished Alumni Achievement Service Award on him in 2012. He lives in Seattle, Washington.

Into the Storm

JOURNEYS WITH ALZHEIMER'S

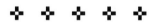

Collin Tong

Editor

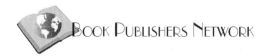

BOOK PUBLISHERS NETWORK

Book Publishers Network
P.O. Box 2256
Bothell • WA • 98041
Ph • 425-483-3040
www.bookpublishersnetwork.com

10 9 8 7 6 5 4 3 2 1
Printed in the United States of America

LCCN 2013956581
ISBN 978-1-940598-18-5

Editor: Julie Scandora
Cover design: Laura Zugzda
Interior design: Leigh Faulkner

A major portion of the author's royalties from the sale of this book will be donated to the Linda Tong Endowed Memorial Scholarship at the University of Redlands.

In Memory Of

Linda D. Tong
(1947–2011)

Contents

Foreword

My father was a salesman. His dream growing up was to be an electrical engineer, but he ran out of money for school after one year at the local junior college, so he settled into a career as close as he could get to his chosen profession. He started selling appliances, then over the years, moved to increasingly more sophisticated tools of the electrical trade—from bells and buzzers to hotel fire alarms and nurses' call systems.

Pop was a terrific salesman. My mom, in the vernacular of the day, used to say he "could sell icemakers to Eskimos." In 1956, Pop won a national sales award. I was nine at the time, so I don't remember what the award was for, but I do remember that one of the proudest moments in Pop's life was standing beside his prize—a brand new Buick *Roadmaster*—in the ballroom of the Fairmont Hotel in San Francisco.

Pop is nearly ninety-eight now, and for many years, he has been for me the face of Alzheimer's disease. He is a slight, gentle, confused man, thankfully still at peace, near—but not yet at—the end of his life. When I asked him last week what he wants for Christmas, he unhesitatingly and enthusiastically replied—a Buick! He's getting a sweater.

My colleague, Collin Tong, honors me by asking me to provide a foreword for his forthright and enlightening anthology, *Into the Storm: Journeys with Alzheimer's Disease.* The arc of our lives has once again brought us together. Nearly fifty years ago, we graduated from neighboring—and rival—San Francisco high schools. My father now lives in an adult family home in Seattle, just down the hall from where Linda, the love of Collin's life, lived and died.

Like him, Kevan Atteberry, Ann Hedreen, Esther Altshul Helfgott, Connie Thompson, and all the passionate and purposeful contributors to *Into the Storm*, I too am a caregiver. Each of us is or has been on a journey with someone we love dearly, a journey we were not prepared to take to a place we would do anything in our power to avoid.

Along with over fifteen million Americans, we are a family of caregivers, united—not only by our anxiety, frustration, and shared dread destiny—but by our determination, humor, mutual respect and affection. I invite you to come *Into the Storm* with us. I believe you will be informed and inspired by the stories, tears, laughter, and abiding love.

Bob Le Roy, Executive Director
Western and Central Washington State Chapter
Alzheimer's Association

Preface

In our aging society, many of us will soon face the daunting task of caring for a family member or loved one with a debilitating illness. Whether it involves caring for an ailing parent, spouse, sibling, or partner, the burden of caregiving exacts an emotional toll on family members and friends alike.

Caregivers whose responsibility it is to care for loved ones with Alzheimer's disease and dementia face especially formidable challenges. Not the least of those is what Dr. Pauline Boss terms the stress and grief associated with ambiguous loss.

"Ambiguous loss is a loss that is unclear," she writes. "It has no resolution, no closure ... The duality of your loved one's being absent and present at the same time is confusing, and finding meaning (or making sense of your situation) becomes immensely challenging. Without meaning, it is hard to cope. It's hard to manage even your day-to-day responsibilities. Ambiguous loss ruptures your relationship as you knew it."[1]

---

[1] Pauline Boss, *Loving Someone Who Has Dementia: How to Find Hope While Coping With Grief and Stress* (San Francisco: Jossey-Bass, 2011), 1-2.

Not surprisingly, recent studies have shown that individuals who care for those with memory loss face unusually high levels of emotional stress. More than one-third report symptoms of depression. Owing to the physical and emotional toll of caregiving, Alzheimer's caregivers had $9.1 billion in additional health care costs of their own in 2012.[2]

In this anthology, caregivers across the United States share their stories of heartache and struggle. Notwithstanding the inevitable setbacks, the writers profiled convey wisdom and resilience. Their testimonies provide a road map for families embarking on the caregiving journey ahead of them.

Shortly after my late wife, Linda, was diagnosed with younger-onset Alzheimer's disease in 2005, I joined a caregivers support group through the Western and Central Washington State Chapter of the Alzheimer's Association. For five years, my participation with the group proved to be a life-giving experience. At the heart of that journey was storytelling, sharing our stories of what being a caregiver is about.

Stories help us navigate life's complex problems. They provide self-understanding that can illumine some of our most intractable dilemmas. As a character in Peter Shaffer's play *Equus* famously said, stories help us to see more clearly in the dark.[3] Hearing how other individuals tackled the challenges of juggling work and caregiving, often at considerable risk to their own emotional and physical health, was fortifying.

At a deeper level, stories enable us to reframe our human predicament. Thus sharing our narratives creates an atmosphere in which new possibilities for effective caregiving are more clearly revealed. Quaker theologian and educator Parker Palmer wisely observed, "When truth is told through the imaginative patterns of stories and poems, we have a chance

---

[2] Alzheimer's Association, 2013 Alzheimer's Disease Facts and Figures, *Alzheimer's & Dementia, Vol. 9, Issue 2.*

[3] Peter Shaffer, *Equus* (New York: Penguin Plays, 1984).

to be caught up and rewoven into truth's own designs."[4] In that sense, we are re-membered.

Yet even as this book casts a light on the quandaries of ambiguous loss, it is not a how-to book that offers easy formulas. Life circumstances invariably differ, and the very complexities of caregiving defy simple prescriptions. One thing the many contributors to this anthology do agree on, however, is that a network of support is crucial for self-care.

My own support group buoyed me over the course of my own wife's prolonged illness. At the time that Linda first developed Alzheimer's more than fifteen years ago, I knew little about the disease. Hearing the real-life experiences of my fellow caregivers taught me how to be more effective. Their tales of exemplary fortitude spawned the idea for this book.

Like a support group, these stories provide a kaleidoscope of helping voices from individuals facing different life challenges and sharing their personal reflections. Its breadth supplements the many fine memoirs that document the experiences of individual caregivers. In collecting those testimonies, it was my intent to present a multiplicity of individual perspectives on caregiving that reaches out to people everywhere. Thus, I sought stories that are not airbrushed but, rather, articulate the real-life frustrations of people helping their loved ones.

They include a mother (and daughter) caring for her divorced sixty-year-old husband, a married couple in St. Louis coping with the multiple trauma of providing support for four parents who later succumbed to Alzheimer's, a gay man whose partner (a retired Roman Catholic priest) develops the disease, an African American television journalist in Seattle who takes a train to Portland every month to look after an eighty-six-year-old mother suffering from dementia, and a Boston psychotherapist's moving tale of her seventy-two-year-old husband

---

[4] Parker Palmer, *The Active Life: Wisdom for Work, Creativity, and Caring* (San Francisco: Harper Collins, 1990), 11.

(a former professor of comparative literature) whose Alzheimer's diagnosis challenges them to live the spiritual teachings they had embraced in their life together.

An estimated 5.2 million Americans of all ages had Alzheimer's disease in 2013. That includes about five million people age sixty-five and older and approximately two hundred thousand individuals younger than age sixty-five who have younger-onset Alzheimer's. Worldwide, more than thirty-five million people now live with the condition, and that number is expected to double by 2030 and more than triple by 2050 to 115 million.

Last year, more than 15.4 million families and friends provided 17.5 billion hours of unpaid care to those with Alzheimer's and other dementias.[5] For those caregivers especially, a community of care can be life sustaining. Reclaiming a sense of agency in relationship with a broader network of caregivers on that same journey is the ultimate aim of this book.

Caregiving stories also reveal something about the relationship between struggle and hope, and the resiliency of the human spirit. "Life forges us in struggle," Joan D. Chittister reminds us. How we deal with adversity has everything to do with the very measure of ourselves. The unique challenges facing caregivers, in particular, are an invitation to change and growth. "It is not struggle that defeats us ... [but] our failure to struggle that depletes the human spirit."[6]

It is my hope that these stories will provide support for the millions of families embarking on this long road of caregiving and solace in the knowledge that they are not alone.

Collin Tong
January 2014

---

[5] Alzheimer's Association, 2013 Alzheimer's Disease Facts and Figures, *Alzheimer's & Dementia*, Vol. 9, Issue 2.

[6] Joan D. Chittister, *Scarred by Struggle, Transformed by Hope* (Grand Rapids, Michigan: William B. Eerdmans Publishing Company, 2003), 2–3.

In the deserts of the heart
Let the healing fountain start.

- W. H. Auden

Part One

The Ambiguity of Loss

Halfway along the road of this our life
I woke to find myself in a wood so dark
That straight and honest ways were gone,
And light was lost.

– Dante

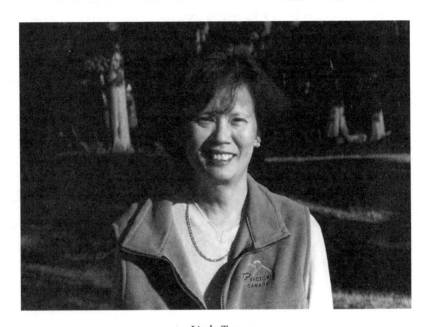

Linda Tong

1

A Caregiver's Notebook

COLLIN TONG[1]

It was more than fifteen years ago, in 1999, when I first discovered that my wife was having serious problems with short-term memory. We were on a walking tour of Provence in southern France when I noticed that Linda had forgotten to bring several items for our vacation.

After we arrived in Paris, we spent a half-day wandering around the city looking for stores to buy contact lens solution, sunscreen, toothpaste, a face cloth, and other sundries.

I didn't think anything was amiss until we returned to Seattle that October. Unanticipated events had dealt us a major blow when her younger sister, who had recently had a kidney transplant, died from complications during a routine dialysis. Linda's memory lapses only increased during her protracted grieving process.

---

[1] "A Caregiver's Notebook" was adapted from an article, "My Journey with Alzheimer's Disease," published in the *Seattle Post-Globe* (November 15, 2009), and is reprinted with permission.

Coworkers noticed that Linda was having more difficulty at Seattle City Light where she had worked for twenty years as an energy conservation analyst. A normally well-organized person, she forgot her appointments and drove colleagues to distraction by endlessly repeating questions.

This was the same Linda who had been so meticulous about gardening, cooking, taking care of the family finances, and just about every aspect of our forty years together as a married couple. She was always upbeat, vivacious, with an effervescent gleam in her eyes, and the smile that won my heart when we first met in 1971.

Linda took an extended leave of absence so that I could take her to see a neurologist, clinical psychologist, and other dementia specialists. All had reached the same conclusion, namely, that her short-term memory loss stemmed from clinical depression, a diagnosis that later proved to be incorrect.

I continued my communications job at Washington State University and put Linda's memory problems in the back of my mind. I didn't realize it at the time, but I was in denial and slow to face the dreaded possibility that she might be suffering from something more consequential than depression. Indeed, I was only living through the stages of grieving itself: denial, despair, frustration, and increasing isolation from family, friends, and even the person I was caring for.

My normal way of dealing with terminal illness was not to deal with it. Like many people who care for a loved one with dementia, I knew little about Alzheimer's and was hesitant to learn more. I went to bookstores to scan medical books about the disease, but the more I read, the less hopeful I became for any improvement in Linda's condition.

The daily press of work left me little time to focus on her disability. Instead, I took on additional responsibilities, which was a way of coping with the demands of her slow but irreversible deterioration. My mother in San Francisco had died two years earlier of pancreatic cancer, and I was still in the throes of mourning her death.

As time went on, Linda's behavior grew more erratic. Our lives became more challenging as her grief over the passing of her sister continued unabated. Overburdened by the demands of work and caregiving, I took early retirement from my university job.

My growing acceptance of Linda's memory problems notwithstanding, I could not ignore the signs of her cognitive decline. By then, our familiar world was slowly dissolving. She was fifty-seven years old in 2005 when she was diagnosed with early-onset Alzheimer's disease. The news devastated our families and friends. Our lives were about to change profoundly.

Shortly after her diagnosis, I called the Alzheimer's Association 24/7 Helpline in Seattle and spoke with a very helpful staff employee, Karl Thunemann. Karl and I soon realized that we had been reporter colleagues at the *Eastside Journal-American* newspaper in Bellevue many years ago. But his dedication to assisting Linda and me through our unexpected life crisis was obvious long before either of us realized we had a connection.

The physical and emotional toll of being a full-time caregiver is daunting. However much I tried, nothing adequately prepared me for the challenges of 24/7 caregiving. I felt overwhelmed with the daily chores of cooking, cleaning, shopping, paying bills, mowing the lawn, doing the laundry, or just attending to the daily necessities of keeping our lives afloat.

We went to church less frequently, began skipping social activities, and even did the unthinkable, missed my nephew's wedding in California. Our friends felt our absence all the more keenly because we had been so active in the community before Linda's debilitating illness.

Fortunately, our families in the San Francisco Bay Area and southern California helped us tackle the financial, legal, and related issues, such as helping Linda to secure her Social Security disability and retirement pension. Linda's brother and family spent a week with her when I attended my Peace Corps reunion in New York.

Friends brought over hot meals and cared for Linda whenever I ran errands, visited friends, or needed a break. One retired couple helped mend a broken fence, fix a leaky faucet, and organize our disheveled home. Another bought a new carpet. Our church organized a weekend work party to mow the lawn and beautify our weed-strewn garden. Still another even helped with more mundane tasks, like doing our laundry.

Through trial and error, I learned that, while being a caregiver is challenging, help is always available if one is intentional about seeking it. One only has to reach out to others.

Self-care is of utmost importance. Going out to lunch with friends, seeing a Mariners game, or just taking a walk was replenishing. Equally important is developing a strong network of supportive friends. Fortunately, our friends and church in Seattle, as well as the Alzheimer's Association, became our lifelines.

Most important of all for me was accepting the inevitable feelings of grief and loss as Linda changed and acknowledging the things that were beyond my control while making decisions about things I could control.

At the encouragement of a social worker friend, I joined an early-onset Alzheimer's support group in Seattle. Additionally, the association helped put us in touch with a placement specialist to find an adult family home located less than ten minutes away from our home in the Sunset Hill neighborhood of Ballard. The association has become an integral part of our support system.

Sadly, ours is not a unique experience. More and more people under sixty-five, baby boomers, are getting younger-onset Alzheimer's disease. At last count, Washington State had more than 110,000 people with Alzheimer's. About 70 percent of those individuals live at home, and unpaid caregivers, mostly family and friends, care for 70 percent.

Because of the unrelenting demands of 24/7 caregiving, taking good care of one's physical and emotional well-being is all too often given short shrift. Stress and anxiety inevitably lead to social isolation and the downward spiral of frustration, despair, and hopelessness.

Fortunately, many organizations exist that provide respite care. I helped enroll Linda at an adult day health program in Seattle, where skilled and dedicated care professionals engaged her in daily social interaction that helped maintain her health. Some thirty-six adult day health centers offer services throughout Washington State. In King County alone, they serve about 1,400 elderly and disabled citizens.

Organizations, such as Volunteers of America, also provide invaluable respite care services. In many instances, I turned to friends and family for assistance with taking care of Linda when I needed to take time out from caregiving.

In the final three months of her life, Linda's condition took a precipitous turn for the worse. Following several weeks under the care of hospice workers, she died peacefully after a brave twelve-year struggle on April 5, 2011, surrounded by family and friends in her adult family home just a few hours shy of her sixty-fourth birthday.

Navigating the challenges of caring for a loved one with dementia or Alzheimer's disease need not be a solitary journey. Indeed, as I learned, it is impossible to surmount those hurdles without reaching out to others. Because of our extended network of family and friends who went the extra mile to be our lifelines and safety net, ours has been a life-transforming and life-affirming journey.

2

Northern House

ANN HEDREEN[1]

Trying to find a home for someone who's done a stint at the Seattle Geropsychiatric Center is like trying to find a home for a paroled sex offender. We weren't yet accustomed to thinking of our mother as a parolee, an ex-con of the dementia world.

So we were grateful for Northern House.

Lynette, the Geropsych social worker, labored hard to find this new address for Mom. But that didn't mean we didn't notice things, like the split-level, floor-plan-in-a-can dreariness of the place; the peeling, Kleenex-blue paint; the faint lines of moss creeping up the outside walls; the cloying floral furniture you wouldn't wish on your most impoverished college-aged nephew.

Mom loved good woods, strong stripes, and straight lines. She would never have chosen Northern House in a million years.

---

[1] "Northern House" is excerpted from Ann Hedreen's *Her Beautiful Brain* (Berkeley, CA: She Writes Press, 2014) and is reprinted with permission.

And yet, it was surrounded by tall trees, some of them probably 150 years old, big, patient, second-growth Douglas firs miraculously left standing when the split-level people came through forty or fifty years ago. And it was tucked into a winding ravine in a neighborhood just north of the Seattle city limits, not too far from the little red ranch house that she and Dad bought when they were newlyweds. Sometimes I took the old highway to get there instead of the freeway and drove past landmarks Mom would have loved: Highland Ice Arena, where she, who had grown up skating in Butte, held out her hands and coaxed us away from the edge of the rink; Leilani Lanes, where she dropped off baby Lisa and me in the upstairs nursery and I watched her through the big glass window, looking so serious as she stared at those pins and then twirling into her huge, happy smile after the crash of a strike, which I still think is one of the best noises in the world.

The round-the-clock staff at Northern House radiated calm and kindness and tree-like patience. Most of them were from Gambia or Ethiopia, and you got the feeling that taking care of people with brain damage and dementia was a breeze compared to some of the earlier chapters of their lives.

They had a completely new view of Mom: the view of people who had never known her any other way.

Before Seattle Geropsych, in her two years at the Lakeview Retirement Community, she had gone from hosting illicit wine parties and modeling at the annual fashion show to yelling at the staff when they tried to call her out of her room for meals and flat-out refusing to bathe. But the caregivers at Northern House had not seen any of that transformation. Nor had they seen her tied to a wheelchair in the Geropsych dayroom. They only knew her as the gnomish white-haired woman who walked up and down the hallway all day, muttering and gesturing but never tiring herself enough to sleep; who looked closer to ninety than she did to her real age, seventy;

who had four blue-eyed daughters who were impossibly hard to keep straight. They didn't wince at having to cut up her food and feed her with a spoon because they didn't know that just a few months ago she'd been feeding herself just fine. They didn't mind if she yelled through her shower because they knew she'd be calm afterwards, soothed by the warm towel and the brush running through her bobbed hair. Arlene didn't have the thatchy old-lady hair of the other women at Northern House: hers was as fine and straight as her many daughters'.

Through the looking glass of a disastrous fall followed by a zombifying dose of anti-psychotic medication and the slow detox at Seattle Geropsych, Mom had slipped into the late stage of Alzheimer's. Outings were now too exhausting and overwhelming. My sisters and I no longer got to play the role of liberators, signing her out for family birthday parties or walks or restaurant meals. Now we were visitors. We brought chocolate and photos and flowers from our gardens. We emailed each other constantly, comparing notes about when we planned to visit so that Mom would have visitors on as many different days as possible and then sending updates about how she was doing when we saw her.

"Anyway, re: my Mom visit last Sat., she seemed OK, much the same. She was very talkative, almost non-stop with a mix of pure gibberish, words that made no sense, and little snippets of meaningful conversation ..."

"So like a baby now it amazes me. She enjoys eating so much ..."

I often came at lunchtime because feeding her gave me something to do. Sometimes, she was happy to see me. Other times, she didn't seem to know me. Sometimes, she liked it when I sat next to her on the couch and put my arm around her as if I was a teenage boy and she was my girlfriend. Sometimes, she liked it when I sang songs, the oldest songs I could think of, songs I remembered her father singing, like "Oh My Darling

Clementine." Whether she was treating me like a daughter or a stranger on any particular day did not seem to have anything to do with how well she liked my cuddling or my laughable singing or the food I was feeding her.

She grew tired and cranky if I stayed too long. At least that's what I told myself, as I watched the clock tick while I sang, talked, spooned macaroni, all the while feeling like some kind of desperate performance artist who just couldn't get the audience to wake up and was now counting the minutes until I could run from the stage. *Herring boxes without topses / Sandals were for Clementine ...*

Maybe my sisters and I shouldn't have been so strict about not visiting on the same days. But we knew that if we were there at the same time, we would be tempted just to talk to each other and ignore Mom and also that it would mean she might not get a visitor on another day. Northern House was not a quick drive for any of us: twenty-five or thirty minutes each way for Caroline or me; an hour and a half each way for Lisa or Kristie.

And, we reasoned, it was good for Mom in a general sense if the staff knew that one of us might stroll in any old time.

What we didn't know is how much of any of it mattered to Mom.

There are so many kinds of loneliness. There's the eerie isolation of being packed into a subway or walking down a crowded street where no one dares to make eye contact. Or the pressing in of the walls when you're alone in a new town and have no one to call. But I've never felt as lonely in all my life as I did when I visited my mother at Northern House. To sit across the table from the person who was the very first person I loved, the very first person to love me; to try with all my might to will her eyes to meet mine and then to have to give up, to accept her eyes not seeing me—and then to have one of her well-meaning caregivers comment on how pretty Arlene looks today, her lovely skin, her clean white hair. I wanted to shout, Who cares? She's gone! Can't you see that this is not Arlene? This is an old-woman rag doll who we are all pretending is still a living person. Can't you see that the reason I have to leave the very minute the clock strikes the hour is not that I have so much work to do, which is what I always say, but because I have to get in my car and drive down the street until I'm out of your sight and then I can stop and let out this sob I've been strangling on for the last half hour?

This went on for four years.

Each visit another downhill step, another bit of bad news to report: she won't chew her food. We have to put her in a diaper. She won't stand up straight. She won't stand up at all. Four years: from walking and muttering to limp and mute in a wheelchair, all connections between brain and muscles severed.

And during those four years, the visits to Mom were sandwiched between all the rest of my life, just as they were for my sisters and for my brother when he visited from New Jersey. Sandwiched. It sounds so easy, a simple matter of tucking the ham in-between the bread and the lettuce. But it never was. It was never easy to tuck a known mood-wrecker into the day, to know that I was going to get up from my desk, get in my car, and drive into a wall, again, and then recover, again, like the world's most resilient crash-test dummy. It was never easy to do it, not knowing how many months or years I was going to keep doing it, which meant I couldn't have a big breakdown every time; I just couldn't. It wouldn't be fair to my husband or children or friends or workmates.

So I learned what I needed to do to smother the sadness and get on with the day. I stopped for the sob down the block from Northern House, and then, if I had time, I did some transitional something between the visit with Mom and having to function in the world of my daily life. If I had time, I went to Third Place Books, over the hill from Northern House. If I felt too wrecked to browse books, I would browse magazines in their café over a bowl of soup, a practice the store graciously allowed. There were a few friends I could walk with or have lunch with immediately after visiting Mom, and I could either talk about her or not.

But there were many people I felt I could not see or talk to right after seeing her. My dad and stepmom, for example. They couldn't help being healthy and athletic and youthful; it was irrational of me to think of their good fortune as somehow unfair. But here they were, flying back and forth to Phoenix for their tennis and golf and sunshine while Mom lived out her shredded life at Northern House. And here I was, that old divorce scar tissue flaming up whenever Dad asked, "How's Arlene?" I knew it made no sense. And yet it was true.

Maybe all grave illnesses do this to families: bring up old hurts, inflame old wounds. But Alzheimer's disease has its own particularly insidious torture methods. One is the open-endedness of it. There is no three-month, six-month, couple-of-years-if-you're-lucky kind of diagnosis as you might get with cancer. It could be a year or a decade. Or two decades. Mom's body was strong. So I couldn't afford not to tamp down the sadness after my visits.

I had to conserve emotional energy.

Another of Alzheimer's tortures is that once you've passed a certain point, you can no longer talk about it with the person who has it. There is no crying together about the awfulness of fate; there are no good-byes. If Mom was raging against her illness somewhere deep inside, we didn't know it. She couldn't tell us.

I wondered often, at Northern House, if she was. Raging. If her pacing and muttering and later, in the wheel-chair, her sudden bursts of incoherent agitation were her ways of trying to say, Why? Why can't you get me out of here, out of this canyon, this cavern? Why can't someone or something or some drug get in here and clear a path through my brain?

She was so helpless, so lost. Watching her, we were too. *Lost and gone forever / Dreadful sorry, Clementine.*

3

Shifting Gears

CONNIE THOMPSON

It's Saturday morning, 7:30 a.m., as my train pulls out of the King Street Station in Seattle for the three-and-a-half-hour trip south to Portland—my quiet before the changing of the guard.

It has become a monthly ritual. Either by train or car, I shift gears from being a full-time television journalist, wife, and domestic operations manager to a respite provider for my sister and caregiver for our eighty-six-year-old-mother, Betty. Thanks to my sister's sacrifice and dedication, my mother still lives at home. My sister also works full time, so we're both exhausted as the weekend begins.

By my calculations, dementia started creeping into Mom's life, and ours, in the mid-nineties. She held her own as a widow on social security and managed well with her independence. Highly intelligent and active in the community, my mother was recognized as a pioneering leader and civic affairs advocate in Portland.

At some point in her late sixties or early seventies, however, we started to notice subtle changes in her behavior.

She began to repeat sentences, left bills unpaid, withdrew from others, and used her finely-tuned coping skills to mask her growing memory loss. Denial was a soothing prescription for all of us—until it stopped working.

The turning point for me came early one August after I had spent a weekend in Portland. We had driven to Costco, for what I can't recall. This was back when Mom was still present enough to stay home (and nap if she chose) or go along for the ride. Shortly after dropping her off at the house, I prepared to shift gears and start the 168-mile drive back to Seattle. "Call when you get home!" she said. When I called, Mom picked up the phone. "It's Connie, Mom. I'm home."

"That's good. How was the drive?" she asked.

"It was fine. What are you doing?" I replied.

"Just piddling, I guess," she said. "I don't know. I went somewhere with someone earlier."

"That was me, Mom. We went to Costco. I was just down to see you. Don't you remember?"

The conversation escalated into a tearful argument as I begged her to see a doctor and have her memory checked because we were concerned. Although Mom defiantly insisted that there was nothing wrong with her memory, I tried to convince her that I didn't want her to be exploited like so many victims of consumer fraud that I report about. She tearfully urged me not to cry because she was fine. Thanks to the Alzheimer's Association, my family would later learn that high-stress arguing is not a constructive approach when you're communicating with someone whose memory is impaired.

I often wonder how things might have worked out if Dad were still alive. Our family has always been close, and there are few challenges we've not been able to cope with together. As our mother used to remind us, "Can't never did anything." I parrot that phrase to her and to myself with regularity now, as we encounter situations that make each of us feel we can't go on.

From time to time, I've threatened my mother that I would one day write a book based on her now family-famous quotes. She used them frequently when I was growing up. "Hard times will make a monkey eat red peppers!" she'd quip at our protests against certain foods we did not want to eat. Childhood fits of anger would be met with "When you get mad, you just have to get glad!"

Mom's quotes were the source of countless jokes. Now, decades later, those simple sayings are our source of strength as our mother surrenders her once-brilliant mind to dementia. I wish you could have known her back then, but I'd be proud for you to meet her today, shredded short-term memory and all. You'd be charmed by Betty Thompson and the spark that still burns from within to remind you "I'm still here!"

Juggling the demands of caring for a loved one with Alzheimer's or dementia can tear a family apart. So I'm thankful that my sisters and I recognized early on that the best way to help our mother would be to acknowledge the obvious and work together. So many families stay in denial until it's too late. The three best things we ever did were to contact the local Alzheimer's Association for resources and support, get Mother a new and more qualified physician, and commit to putting aside our sibling differences and agree that Mom's care and well-being come first.

The sudden death of our brother in 2000 plucked away a vital member of our family caregiving team just as Mom's short-term memory loss was becoming impossible to ignore. We knew we were in trouble when Mom stopped. She stopped answering the phone, answering the door, calling her friends, attending club meetings and social events; she even stopped going to church.

Mom stayed awake every night with the television as her companion and slept during the day. With our father and brother gone and a younger sister battling cancer in California, it fell to my Portland sister to become Mom's primary caregiver. My sister eventually stored most of her belongings and moved back home to the bedroom we once shared as kids. Her life as a full-time caregiver has been the ultimate test of her strength.

Life took an unexpected turn shortly after Easter in 2001 when I received a phone call from my sister. She had come home from running an errand to find the heat turned up high and the house full of steam. Mom was in the bathtub, flat on her back, her head perilously close to submerging, and struggling to breathe with the tub filling up with hot water. Doctors would later diagnose a problem with her heartbeat, a sign that she also might have suffered a mini-stroke.

Mom spent three weeks in intensive care, the first nine days with a breathing tube down her throat. Taking shifts almost around the clock at the hospital, my two sisters and I were told to "get things in order." We signed the DNR (Do Not Resuscitate) documents and said many prayers. We were prepared for the worst, but Mom came out of it. After a month of rehabilitation, she was back home with a double pacemaker. But she did not remember a thing about what had happened.

After that episode, while Mom was still able to make decisions, she appointed me Power of Attorney. My Portland sister was the obvious choice to handle all medical decisions. Thank God. In the ensuing years, the dementia has accelerated its march through Mom's brain, leaving Swiss cheese holes in her short-term memory. Her body, meanwhile, works just fine.

Many people fail to realize that you can have Alzheimer's or dementia and be aware of the fact. My mother knows she can't remember. She struggles with not knowing what's going on. As heartbreaking as it is to see your loved one's mental capacity diminish, it's almost torture to hear that loved one talk to herself about losing her mind.

"I just don't understand why God isn't ready for me," I heard Mom mumble one Sunday. "I'm of no use," she said. "I have no purpose. You get old, and everyone tells you what to do. You can't remember anything. You lose control of your life."

As caregivers, my sister and I try to stay mindful of the fact that we have taken control of virtually every aspect of our mother's life—and we must do that with respect. The part of her that is still here wants to have a say about what she does, so whenever possible, we give her choices. Would you prefer spaghetti or chicken soup? Do you want to wear the blue outfit or the green?

We also try to include her in conversations and let her know her knowledge and opinions are valued. Can you help me add the charges on this bill? What do you think about painting the house purple? Would you like to use the bathroom before you lie down? Sure, we already know the answers. The point is Mom is engaged and included rather than always being told what to do and where to go. It makes a difference by reducing the stress and giving her back at least some of the control.

You'll often hear that caregiving for someone with memory loss can be like taking care of a baby. It's true. Some call it a forty-eight-hour day. We have many light moments with warm laughs and traces of the family times we once had before dementia. But mostly, it's hard work. And you never know when it's about to get more difficult.

Two days after a pleasant family Christmas 2011 in Portland, Mom fell and fractured her pelvis. My husband and I got the call from our nephew while on the train back home to Seattle. Time to switch gears again.

A week in traction in the hospital was followed by a five-week nightmare at a skilled rehabilitation nursing facility. Many facilities claim to have memory-care expertise, but I'm skeptical. In our case, my stressed-out mother was petrified, in extreme pain, and to a large degree, dismissed. Fortunately our family remained diligent and involved—juggling our schedules and enlisting friends to help take shifts so someone was on hand to help and reassure Mother almost 24/7. We slept in an old reclining chair, watched the staff like hawks, answered Mom's constant questions, and took copious notes. You can't select care facilities in a hurry, and you can't expect any facility to give your loved one the level of care you would provide.

If you're lucky in this situation, you have the help, finances, good information, and resources to guide you through the maze of insurance companies, home health services, case-workers, private care services, transport services, doctors, and medical equipment specialists. Often, however, you are alone and get conflicting information or no information. If you don't know what you're doing or whom to ask, the system alone can drive you insane. The pressure and stress drive some people to just take off. So we know we're lucky. And so far we're still afloat.

For as long as we can swing it, the private-pay care-givers and adult care center will give my sister and Mom the added support they need. These days, while I'm at work or at home in Seattle, I keep my personal phone at the ready, just in case. I worry that at any time the phone will ring with bad news. I worry about how long my sister can keep it up without cracking, or worse. My sisters and I gather information and resources that can help us help Mom the best we can.

I don't know how much longer my mother will live. Although her dementia continues to worsen, her little body keeps on going like the Energizer Bunny. I don't know how long my sisters and I will be able to hang in there—financially, phys-ically, or emotionally. Whenever I look at my mother's sweet smile and she hugs us and says, "You're wonderful daughters," I realize what a gift it is to be caring for her and honoring the lesson she taught us—that life itself is a precious gift, regardless of the circumstances.

That isn't to say I don't feel overwhelmed, exhausted, or sad at how Mother's life turned out. But as Mom often reminds us, "Expectations and reality are often two different things." And so, with love and gratitude I count my blessings, take a deep breath, and prepare to switch gears and get back on the road.

4

Dying with Mom—and Living

ARLENE ZAREMBKA

My mother was a brilliant woman, a math major when she attended college in the thirties. She minored in physics and astronomy, but her real passions were Shakespeare and grand opera. I had always been very close to her. When I was twenty-eight, I moved back to St. Louis to practice law and be closer to my parents. As the in-town adult child, I enjoyed spending time with them. I could scarcely have imagined that I would one day become both a caregiver and "parent" to my mother.

Mental acuity was always important to Mom. Convinced that alcohol would destroy her brain cells, she remained a life-long teetotaler. The thought that she would eventually succumb to Alzheimer's disease herself never crossed my mind. Never, that is, until I witnessed her first memory lapse.

For my Christmas present in 1988, she gave me the identical book that my partner, Zuleyma, had given me for my birthday less than two months earlier (a biography of Janusz Korczak, the renowned Polish-Jewish pediatrician who perished in Treblinka). Mom had even exclaimed what a perfect birthday present it was since it was about my father's native Poland and the Holocaust, a strong shared interest of ours.

Initially, Mom's short-term memory glitches were infrequent, and she knew how to disguise them by saying the socially appropriate thing. Zuleyma and I weren't always certain if she was actually having a memory lapse or if it was just our imagination. By 1991, however, Mom was beginning to show unmistakable signs of forgetfulness. She stopped studying Japanese, for example, because she could no longer remember the *kanji* words (Chinese characters used in Japanese writing) that she looked up.

While it was apparent to her St. Louis family—Dad, Zuleyma, and me—that her memory was getting worse, Mom sounded normal when she talked by phone to my three out-of-town siblings. Because they could not fully grasp the unfolding tragedy of Mom's profound memory loss, a chasm of misunderstanding opened up between us.

By 1993, Dad and I managed to get her to agree to a geriatric assessment, couching it as a routine evaluation. Mom's mental abilities remained above average. The geriatric assessment team was unable to determine whether her short-term cognitive impairment was irreversible and thought that her poor eating habits might be the real cause of her decline. The fact that Mom was eating so poorly shocked us, as she had always made good nutritious home meals.

A month later, Mom began talking unintelligible gibberish. The doctor diagnosed pneumonia and admitted her to the hospital. Despite improvements to her diet, her memory continued to deteriorate.

Even though I knew she was slipping, I remained in denial about the severity of her dementia. In April 1994, Zuleyma and I returned home late one evening after taking her to a Shakespeare play. As Mom got into her car to drive home, Zuleyma and I watched from our window as she sat motionless in her car in the pouring rain. After many minutes had passed, I went out to the car and noticed she had not turned on the ignition.

When I motioned her to roll down her window, she couldn't remember how to do so. Nor could she recall how to start the ignition with the car key. I am embarrassed to say that I started the car for her and told Mom that home was three miles straight ahead. I went back into the house and called Dad to make sure she made it home safely.

A month later, Mom was hospitalized with pneumonia. Signs of her cognitive impairment began to surface when she began talking unintelligible gibberish. Sometime during that hospital stay, a neurologist diagnosed Mom with Alzheimer's disease. When she returned home, Mom was a changed person. Although her ability to talk understandably had resumed, she now had a flat affect instead of her formerly alert and intelligent face.

With the Alzheimer's diagnosis, it was no longer possible for me to deny that Mom's condition was never to improve. I felt a jumble of emotions—sadness at losing my mother as I had known her, anger at the unknown demon that caused her Alzheimer's, shock that I was reading books about that dreaded, mind-robbing disease, helplessness that I couldn't halt the deterioration of her mind, guilt about the times I had not taken her out, called, or visited or hadn't purchased the *Ginkgo biloba* when she asked me if I could find something to help with her memory problems.

Zuleyma and I soon joined the adult children's support group of the St. Louis chapter of the Alzheimer's Association. The group became our lifeline to sanity over the ensuing eleven years. We quickly found that well-meaning friends, and even siblings, could not provide the same support and practical suggestions that the association and support group provided. Our friends had never been close to someone with Alzheimer's, and my siblings all lived far from us. They did not observe, as we did, the daily changes brought about by Mom's dementia.

Shortly before Mom's diagnosis, the first drug to treat Alzheimer's had come on the market. Dad promptly bought the new medication for Mom. Over the next few weeks, Mom began to lose her appetite and ate less and less. We couldn't convince Dad to call her physician because Dad wanted to wait until her next scheduled visit. He finally agreed that we should call my sister, who is a doctor, and she called Mom.

Mom explained that she had been sick and hadn't felt like eating. She convinced my out-of-town sister that she was fine, but Dad, Zuleyma, and I all knew that Mom still was not eating. Only when her regular doctor stopped the medication did her appetite return.

For the first year after Mom's diagnosis, we didn't know how to "reach" her. Then one day, Zuleyma quoted a well-known poem while driving with Mom. Mom perked up and wanted to repeat the poem. We were elated.

We discovered that Mom could still read poems with meaning and emotion, even though her recollection of the experience was short-lived. Moreover, she remained enraptured by her grand opera and sang "The Star-Spangled Banner" perfectly. We began reading poems with her on a regular basis. Mom and I even took turns reciting portions of Shakespearean plays.

In spite of our newfound connection with Mom, as her descent into Alzheimer's continued unabated, I began to experience growing bouts of depression. I had never been a chronically depressed person and always approached life with enthusiasm and energy. It didn't occur to me that anti-depressants might alleviate my condition. It was not until five years later, a year after Dad died in 1999, that I began taking an anti-depressant, which greatly moderated the depression.

In the meantime, life became increasingly overwhelming. Mom became Dad's shadow, leaving him precious little time to himself. He was in his early eighties and clearly needed assistance with caregiving responsibilities. A fiercely independent man, however, he resisted any help, except from the family. After months of cajoling, he agreed that Mom could go to an adult day-care center three times a week.

Mom put up a fierce resistance, however, and guilt-tripped Dad about sending her away. After two weeks, he threw in the towel and canceled adult day care. For the next six months, Zuleyma and I despaired of ever finding respite for my father. He finally agreed to accept a caregiver for two hours a day, three days a week. Meanwhile, I continued to drown in depression.

By 1997, three years after Mom's diagnosis, I realized that I was dying with Mom but resolved that I had to continue to live. Zuleyma and I began carving out one night a week when we didn't answer the phone or talk about work, Mom's condition, or any other stressful topic. Instead, we made time to read to one another about our favorite subjects, science and history. That break became a welcome respite from our weekly regimen.

In September, we took a wonderfully relaxing vacation to Mexico to visit the Mayan ruins. As soon as I got off the plane, I immediately felt depressed. For the next four months, Zuleyma and I resumed the unrelenting chores of care management for my parents. We missed numerous days at work and took turns getting ill.

By February 1998, I was exhausted and burnt out by the constant stress and depression, as well as Dad's stubborn resistance to common-sense suggestions. Fortunately, my siblings took turns calling him every day to check in, giving Zuleyma and me a much-needed break. That reprieve proved to be all-too short, however, for 1998 turned out to be a year of crisis. In April, Dad fell and broke his thighbone. When we learned that he was in the emergency room, Zuleyma rushed from a conference to be with him. I rushed from my law office to be with Mom so that she would not wander from the house.

I called the homecare agency to arrange 24/7 care for Mom and asked my siblings to come to St. Louis to help out. Zuleyma and I were scheduled to leave in less than two weeks for a long-planned trip to Israel to visit my sister, and I needed to make arrangements for Mom's round-the-clock care. My sister from Israel flew in for a week to assist, and one brother also came in. Two nephews eventually came in, one staying for almost three months.

Shortly after Dad returned home seven weeks later, he sent our nephew home. Notwithstanding his own declining condition, Dad maintained his self-sufficiency. Mom continued to wander, however, and needed more assistance with her daily activities. She also was becoming incontinent. I resumed my caregiving responsibilities.

By December, my eighty-five-year-old father was failing. I alerted my siblings that I thought something would happen in the near future. Early in 1999, Dad began vomiting. As Zuleyma was driving Dad to the doctor, he told her that if he were hospitalized I should put Mom in a nursing home. One of my brothers and I eventually found one that had a memory care unit. Acting as her power of attorney, I signed the paperwork for Mom's admission to the home.

My other brother strongly objected, and the resulting family dissension ripped my life apart. I knew nursing home care was the only realistic option for my mother, given her advanced stage of decline from Alzheimer's. Moreover, my parents had entrusted me to make decisions on their behalf. Shortly before my father's death in early 1999, I admitted Mom to the nursing home, where she lived for the next six years.

Four months after Dad's death, one brother filed a lawsuit seeking guardianship of Mom. My other brother supported his seeking guardianship. Although the suit was unsuccessful, it caused deep divisions in my family. I had lost my father and was losing Mom day by day from Alzheimer's disease. I now lost my relationship with my brothers, as well as the close ties I had with several other family members.

Over the next year as I struggled to put my life back together, knowing that I had chosen a nursing home that was the right place for my mother to live out her final days gave me the strength to endure the "slings and arrows of outrageous fortune." I was there for Mom in her "long goodbye." I built a new life and, over the next several years, restored several family relationships that had been strained by the conflict.

My mother enjoyed a safe and active life at the nursing home until a major stroke in December 2001 left her unable to walk, dance, or enjoy music. She died at age ninety-one in 2005.

5

Alive in New Ways

STEVE KNIPP

My partner, David, and I recently visited Volcano National Park where you learn much about volcanic lava flows, eruptions, and catastrophic destruction of the landscape. The hardened lava creates a new layer of earth and transforms itself into lush fragrant tropics.

This can often be the case in our own lives. David described his own personal volcano to a friend this way: "I have a start of Alzheimer's in my life. It's part of getting older. But I believe we can be alive in new ways."

Alive in new ways? That really struck me. What does it mean for him to be alive in new ways? He puts it this way: "I prefer to accept the things that happen to me. Many things have happened to me during my life, and it's all OK."

Words to live by, for sure.

I grew up in Bay City, Michigan, and moved to Houston, Texas, when I graduated from high school in 1980. I wanted to escape a small town where coming out as a gay man would have been difficult. My first partner and I owned a small real estate company. When his health began to falter, we blamed it on the stress of owning a business. We decided to sell it and move to Seattle to start a new life. When his health didn't improve, we discovered that he had AIDS. My diagnosis came shortly thereafter. My partner died two years later. He was forty-one; I was twenty-nine. We were together for eight years.

I was diagnosed with full-blown AIDS, which meant my immune system was significantly weakened but my health was good. I finished college with a degree in graphic design. But my partner's death still haunted me as did the death sentence that having AIDS in 1991 meant. In trying to cope with the loss, I decided to share my story with those who might be willing to listen. This is how I met my current partner, David. He was a priest and the director of the Catholic AIDS Ministry. He was educating parishioners on the reality of people who were living with AIDS. He also ministered to those affected by the disease. He would invite people with AIDS to tell their stories in parish settings, and I was a member of a panel.

David's short-term memory problems began rather gradually. His general memory loss seemed unremarkable at first but quickly became more pronounced. He couldn't remember words to describe things he had known his whole life. He was always excellent with words and language—he knew Latin, after all. I spoke to my doctor about what I noticed, and she referred us to a neurologist for testing. After months of David not wanting to do this, his memory problems became more and more pronounced, so he finally agreed.

His first neurologist tested him for dementia. In communicating his findings to us, the doctor didn't come right out and say that David had Alzheimer's. Instead, he said, "Yes, there are memory problems, and maybe taking medications will help." I knew what this meant. David didn't pick up on the cues that the doctor gave because the doctor didn't speak directly enough. I went home thinking that David understood, but when I brought up the *A* word, David refused to believe this and continued to deny that he had Alzheimer's.

This made it hard for me to speak openly about David's disease. I called the Alzheimer's Association hotline about my frustration that I couldn't speak with David about his condition. They were helpful and sent loads of information. I began to get more familiar with what we were up against but still felt ill-equipped to know what to do next.

Before David was able to acknowledge this diagnosis, I shared it with his sisters and some of my close friends. This made it hard on his sisters because they were ready to jump in and help. When they learned that David was in denial about his disease, they honored that. It wasn't until nearly six months later that one sister recommended we get a second opinion. This time he understood his diagnosis.

On our visit to the second doctor, she not only tested David but also interviewed me. When she was certain of the diagnosis, she was direct with David: "I think you may already know this, but to be completely clear, the testing we did today confirms without a doubt that you have early-onset Alzheimer's."

The look on David's face was one of complete surprise. He had been in denial—and needed this direct communication to understand. Once David learned of the diagnosis, he was more open about it with his family and friends. He was sixty-five when diagnosed.

I began to seek out support groups and discovered one for the gay community. I have enjoyed getting to know the other members. Sharing provides emotional support. Hearing how others handle issues that you may encounter is helpful. The biggest support group we have lies in David's family, who love and care for him very much. He has three younger sisters, all of whom have stepped up with lots of support as we move into this experience together.

I'm still in the process of figuring out what kinds of planning to do. The hardest challenge now is to balance David's need for independence with the reality that I need to step in and help. This is especially true with financial matters and other tasks that require planning. For instance, David decided to drive to a workshop in an area that he has known his whole life. He asked me for a map with directions. That evening before the event, I glanced at his printed directions and found notes in red ink all over the pages. He did not feel certain about how to get to that familiar place. When I offered to take him, he accepted.

Planning leaves me bewildered because the course of the disease is so different for each person. David still works part-time and is able to take care of himself. How does one plan? We have updated our wills and downsized our living arrangements. Beyond that, I don't know what else can be done. Imagining future scenarios leaves me emotionally exhausted.

Yet for me, the hardest thing is accepting the loss of the man David used to be, of the equal partnership we had. Our communication has changed. We used to have stimulating, intellectual conversations about many topics, but his capacity to follow complex conversations has diminished significantly.

Our recent vacation to Hawaii had me reeling for a few days because I realized on the first day that organizing our day-to-day events was going to fall solely on me. While that may not sound like a big issue, it represented how lopsided our decision making had become. I spent a few days feeling sorry for myself and struggling with how to pull myself together to make the best of the trip. After all, we were in Hawaii!

I recognize that the way we connect has changed. Our relationship is morphing from one of equal partnership to that of caregiver/companion. I've found it difficult to adjust to relating to David in this new way. Being twenty years younger also creates some challenges. Where he seems content to sit home and stick to a routine, I'm still active and pursuing life interests.

I ask myself what is expected of me in this relationship now that it has changed. I love and care about him deeply. I will be as present and supportive as I can be with him through this. Yet it's hard to balance my desire to develop other close, intimate friendships with the reality that David and our relationship are still here. What can I create that honors both of us? At the instinctual level, I know I must pay attention to myself; otherwise, both of us will suffer.

It is reassuring that David is no longer a person in denial. He does not try to hide what has happened to him. Most days he seems happy. He admits to others what is going on. Where he once thrived performing Mass to hundreds of people each week, he now affects people individually by his gentle nature, ready smile, and peaceful presence.

When David and I met twenty years ago, my life expectancy was one to two years. I felt secure that I would be cared for by someone special like him. Then the AIDS medication came out. My death sentence was postponed. Ironically, here we are twenty years later, and I've become the caregiver. Who could have seen this coming?

For those in the caregiving role, something to consider: don't let your beliefs about conventional relationships get in the way of your happiness. At a certain point, you realize that the relationship is no longer the same. It's easy to feel guilt if you start feeling differently about your partner or spouse. Seek out friendships that fill some of gaps in your life. Live your life, ask for help, and chuck conventional wisdom out the window.

As David said, "Be alive in new ways."

6

A Journey through Alzheimer's Country

ESTHER ALTSHUL HELFGOTT

One night in 2005, before Abe went into an assisted living facility, while we were lying in bed, he said, "I never thought that in all my life I would have such a good friend as you." I was taken aback. He said those words with absolute clarity at a time in our lives when he was suffering from aphasia and extreme confusion. "Really?" I said.

He nodded, and we continued lying side by side holding hands until he fell asleep. I watched him as a mother would a newborn child but also as a wife who knew she would not have her partner with her for very much longer. And even then—two or three years into Alzheimer's disease—I felt he was still my partner. Alzheimer's doesn't mean you're dead; it means you're living life differently. Alzheimer's doesn't mean a relationship is dead; it's just changed.

We met in January 1981 at a Seattle congregation. He sat down next to me before an evening class on Conservative Judaism. I was a single parent and a graduate student in history at the University of Washington. He was a single parent and a physician. I was from Baltimore and grew up above a grocery store; he was from the Bronx and grew up behind a grocery store. He had been in Seattle since the 1960s; I arrived in the mid-1970s.

We were two East Coast Jews delighted for cultural and intellectual compatibility. That night, we gabbed until the rabbi came in and gabbed some more after class. We made a lunch date for the following week and met at an old-time restaurant on Capitol Hill, where we continued talking, and continued talking some more, through ups and downs, for the next thirty years. We married in September 1981.

I don't know when Alzheimer's knocked at our door. It was sometime after 2000. In that year, four years after his retirement, Abe had hip-replacement surgery. It seems to me that he never fully recovered. Maybe he already had Alzheimer's and couldn't fight back from the anesthetic. I've heard other people say that their loved ones developed Alzheimer's after hip surgery; but I don't know.

What I do know is that for the next few years until diagnosis, life was a roller coaster of emotions that I rarely understood. In 2003, after a series of tests, Abe was diagnosed with Alzheimer's. The emotions that followed were no less chaotic than those of the previous few years, but at least I had a name for what was happening to Abe and for what the two of us were experiencing—alone and together.

Now, after diagnosis, my role as caregiver was clearly defined. I was in charge of both of us whereas, pre-Alzheimer's, I depended on Abe to take care of me as well—whether going grocery shopping, doing the dishes, or helping me with my bad sense of direction when I was driving us somewhere. I had to give up the idea of his helping me around the house, in the yard, with the grandchildren.

I was in charge of everything, and I hated it. I lived with hating it. All the while, I continued taking care of us. I got through this crazy time by writing. I wanted to record every word Abe said. I didn't know how long he'd be talking in whole sentences, and I had to save as much of him as I could. Plus, this Alzheimer's thing needed to be cornered. It seemed to me that documenting our Alzheimer's experience would not only help me get through those awful days; also, it might provide a map to what was happening to our lives.

I settled in. "This is how we're living now," I told myself. I went to the Alzheimer's Association support groups, which helped a little but not much. I went to a support group from my synagogue, which helped a little but not much. I talked to family and friends, which helped a little but not much. I joined the Alzheimer's Association on-line community where I developed virtual friends, and that helped a lot. But the one thing that really helped me get through the long days and longer nights was writing.

I had an elevator installed in our three-story house to save me from running up and down the stairs looking for Abe, and it did keep him home three years longer. It also created a few humorous and not so humorous incidents. He took a friend up to the fifth floor, which we didn't have. Another time, I found a group of people sitting in our third-floor bedroom. Once Abe tried to open the elevator door while I was inside, the circuit breaker blew, and I had to figure out how to lower the thing and jump off. Fortunately, I was between the second and first floors so I didn't have to jump very far.

Abe liked to walk, but soon he began getting lost in the neighborhood. I had locks installed on the doors so that he'd have to wait for me before going out. He learned how to use his cane to unhook the locks, and the next thing I knew, a neighbor was bringing him home: "I think your husband is lost."

I took him to senior day care, but he didn't like it and would wander off. So they couldn't keep him. Then I hired a caregiver, but that didn't work out either because one day he woke up from a nap, saw a stranger in the house, and thinking we were being robbed, got a knife and chased the caregiver out the door. I blamed myself because I had given him codeine for the severe pain he said he was experiencing.

The wandering increased. One minute he was standing right next to me; the next I got a call from the church up the street. "I just want to rest," he told the woman at the church door. He was on his way to *shul* a block away. I didn't know he had left the house. Fortunately he was wearing the Alzheimer's alert bracelet, but he was soaking wet and confused. The final straw came one winter night when I turned over in bed and no Abe. He wasn't in the house, on the porch, in the yard. It was 1:00 a.m., and I was frantic, not an unfamiliar feeling at that time. I grabbed my coat and ran through the alley like a crazy woman. It was pitch black.

"Abe? Where are you, Abe?" I found him sitting at the bus stop. "Where are you going, sweetheart?"

"To work," he said, and I took him home.

I couldn't take care of him any longer. It wasn't just about his getting lost, as if that weren't enough. He weighed two hundred pounds. I could get him to the shower and dressed, but when he slipped to the floor, I couldn't pick him up.

In August 2006, I found an assisted living facility. It was twelve miles from our house but was supposed to be top of the line. They said they could take care of him until the end. I figured we had enough equity in the house to pay for the facility. But they couldn't take care of him to the end, and the equity was running out. I applied for and received, with some shame, Medicaid. In January 2008, I had Abe transferred to a nursing home, where he was taken care of until his death on June 15, 2010, a day after his eighty-second birthday.

The year and a half Abe was in assisted living, I ran back and forth from home to facility. And I wrote—poems, essays, fragments, anything that came. Now that Abe was no longer living at home, I got lots of advice about how I should live my life. I'll never forget my meeting with an elder care lawyer. He came to our home, sat right across from me at the table that Abe and I had bought together, told me that the best thing I could do was to divorce Abe and get my life back.

He said that I should sell the house and move south of Seattle, where his practice was, so I could be near his office when I needed advice. I was appalled. This lawyer wasn't the only one who mentioned divorce. I was speaking to a *rebbitzen* one day, and nonchalantly, she suggested that divorce under these circumstances was not unheard of.

Friends and family worried. They wanted me to get on with my life. I'm not sure how they expected me to do this. Besides, everyone was missing the point. This was the man who ate popcorn with me at the movies, who held my hand, who took care of me when I was sick, who rubbed my feet, who helped me raise my children, his stepchildren. This was the man whose face I loved—his eyes, his nose, his mouth, his skin. I could still curl up with him in a love seat, Alzheimer's or not. I needed him. He's been gone several years, and I still need him. He's in my soul.

I thought I would stop writing about Alzheimer's after Abe's death, that I would go back to a project I had started years before. I do work on it occasionally, but the passion is gone. Not that Alzheimer's is my passion, but I'm marooned in its territory. I continue writing my blog, "Witnessing Alzheimer's: A Caregiver's View," which I began when Abe went to the nursing home. I've developed a six-week course, "Writing the Alzheimer's Experience: A Caregiver's Workshop," that I teach frequently.

If enough people tell their stories, the reality of Alzheimer's becomes more visible to the outside world, and just possibly, we'll help researchers in their attempts to find a cure. Sometimes I worry that my writing is a betrayal of Abe's privacy; but Abe was my best friend, and I know he would be proud to be helping me tell our story and to help others tell theirs.

Part Two

Family and Relationships

If we commit ourselves to one person for life, this is not, as many people think, a rejection of freedom; rather, it demands the courage to move into all the risks of freedom, and the risk of love which is permanent.

– Madeleine L'Engle

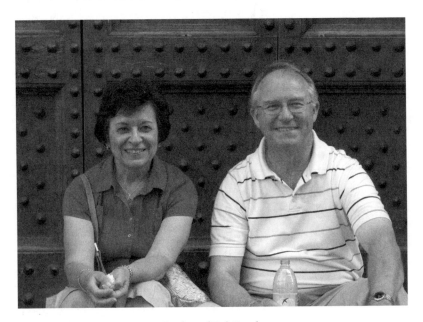

Linda and Bob Brooks

7

Best Friends

BOB BROOKS

In hindsight, nothing could have prepared me for Linda's diagnosis of younger-onset Alzheimer's disease thirteen years ago. Until then, our life together seemed normal. We had been happily married for twenty-four years. She had a long and successful professional career in leadership training, and both of us looked forward to a promising future.

After retiring from a twenty-two-year career in the US Navy, I went to work in the aviation industry teaching aeronautical systems. Shortly thereafter, an international aviation equipment company recruited me to help them start a technical training department. A few years later, the company invited me to serve as its first organizational development specialist.

Linda's family had a history of Alzheimer's disease. Her older sister was diagnosed a few years ago and lives in an Alzheimer's care facility in Massachusetts. While neither of her two older brothers had memory problems, her mother had late-stage Alzheimer's and lived in a care facility until her death in 1991.

Linda's close-knit family seemed the quintessential immigrant success story. Her family heralds from Filicudi, a small Italian island located about twenty miles north of Sicily. As a child, her mother lived in a small house with a dirt floor while her father was a fisherman and, at times, a bricklayer. After World War I, Linda's parents and older brother immigrated to the United States where they built two successful businesses.

After high school, Linda attended secretarial school and landed a job in Boston. Recognizing her greater potential, her supervisor encouraged her to go to college. She took his advice, earned a doctorate in education, and accepted a position with a management consulting firm in Boston. There, Linda was responsible for developing a competency-based leadership-training program for the US Navy.

She eventually parlayed that experience into a management development position for a major West Coast company where she conducted training and designed companywide leadership training programs. Later, she formed and led a training group introducing the company to performance-based training.

Linda's memory problems were slow to develop, and neither of us recognized them to be unusual at the outset. Work seemed to become more difficult and complicated for her. Her company eventually downsized the training group and reassigned her to a satellite station away from company headquarters.

She grew frustrated working below her skill level. At the time, I attributed her forgetfulness and misplaced items to stress at work, corporate politics, or maybe depression. At my urging, she consulted a counselor and received medication, which did not help. Little did we suspect that her memory problems were more serious and deep-seated.

Linda lost her job in 2001. For a couple of years, she worked as a temporary employee while keeping her eye open for better positions. In 2003, she traveled within the United States collaborating with a group of business professionals to write a book for a nonprofit organization. She even started her own business, but working with numbers was daunting, and adapting to new clients and projects became too hard to manage. Soon she avoided looking for new clients and stopped working altogether. It was a depressing and confusing time for her.

We began having loving, though earnest, discussions at home about our mutual expectations. It seemed that Linda was not paying attention during conversations. Trying to compensate for her inattention, I would reach out to touch her arm and make eye contact before I began speaking. We talked about keeping up with our to-do lists. We both needed to remember our plans and commitments.

We agreed to avoid distractions and focus on helping each other. Because I was traveling extensively in my work, I was depending on her to keep everything together at home. Linda apologized for letting me down and promised to do better. But over the coming year, our commitments were to no avail. Neither of us understood that she was no longer able to do these things and could not control what was happening to her.

I encouraged Linda to talk to our doctor again. Again, he told us that everything was normal, but we pushed for more testing. Soon we connected with a doctor who used to work at an Alzheimer's disease research center. He ordered an MRI. He and other doctors examined the images and concluded that her memory and concentration failings were not caused by vascular problems.

Then in November of 2006, we met with a psychologist. The appointment lasted several hours, and as the testing proceeded, Linda began to see the seriousness of the problem. She feared the worst and remembered how her mother and grandmother had struggled with Alzheimer's with no medication and long confinement in a nursing home. That day we received the diagnosis; at age sixty-one, Linda had early onset of Alzheimer's type dementia.

I clearly remember the conversation with the psychologist as she gave me the diagnosis. It felt as if a switch in my head was turned on. In that moment, I realized that the problems with missed appointments, lost items, undone tasks, lack of ambition were not Linda's fault but a result of Alzheimer's disease. Linda could not control what was happening. Linda's diagnosis was heartbreaking for both of us.

We did not understand the mechanics of Alzheimer's but started to learn more about the disease. We talked to people, read books, searched the Internet, and attended workshops. There was no cure, few clues, and little hope. I felt as though we were settling in to live out our lives. The disease would kill Linda, and I would help her travel the path. The more we learned, the more discouraged we became.

At the time of her diagnosis, my employer expected me to move to California. The move promised more money and responsibility, but what would happen at home while I was at the office or on another continent? How would Linda, who had stopped driving, get around in a new environment? How would she develop a new support system, a new circle of friends? How could I make extended trips to other countries for work? Faced with her diagnosis and no answers to our questions, I retired from my job. Within thirty days, I was at home for good.

I began to attend a support group for spouses of younger-onset Alzheimer's patients, which was sponsored by the Alzheimer's Association. I needed to learn how to help my wife and how to cope with the problems ahead. Linda, however, was reluctant to participate. She already knew what she needed to know about the disease. It would be ugly. Lamenting the disease with others seemed to her unproductive.

At first, Linda was uncomfortable telling anyone but close family members about the disease. I told a few of her friends so they could begin understanding and remain available to Linda. She didn't want people to treat her differently because, for her, the disease was private and sharing the news of her disease was an embarrassment. Yet all our friends and family were supportive from the beginning. Linda explains that we don't have any "bad friends."

Neither Linda nor I directly asked for any help from family or friends. But family and friends have stepped forward. My brother and I are close. It's been helpful to explain my frustrations and worries and even some of our laughable Alzheimer's moments. As for Linda, sometimes friends invite her on shopping trips, lunch dates, and chats.

One friend visits several times a week to play Scrabble with her. When I needed to be out of town for a few days, I arranged with friends to visit. They had meals together, went for drives, watched movies, cooked together, and sometimes just sat and talked. Now Linda looks forward to attending support group meetings where she has made new friends.

I did not consciously develop a coping strategy. Linda and I chose each other as best friends, and Alzheimer's disease hasn't changed this part of our relationship. As Linda's short-term memory deteriorates and her cognitive skills wane, I just fill in where I am needed. I have learned to help where I can but not do so much that I rob her of her dignity and autonomy.

It's easy to become frustrated and annoyed with her repeated questions and my endlessly repeated explanations. I still struggle for patience when I explain several times why we need to get out the door and into the car for an appointment while trying to ignore the clock ticking in my head. Despite my years of professional experience working in technical training and organization development, I felt ill-equipped to stay focused during this difficult time.

Although I've always been a well-organized person, caregiving for Linda has presented new challenges. I am getting better at planning ahead, starting sooner, and avoiding last minute changes to our plans. For now, it is enough for me to be a good husband and friend and take one day at a time, to be present and helpful. When it becomes necessary, I will bring in people with new skills and fresher perspectives.

I'm learning to be more conscientious about self-care. I take care of myself through hobbies, study, and exercise. I am aware that if I break down someone else needs to step in to take care of Linda. Finding the right person with the right skills and temperament takes time. A few years ago, we got legal help to articulate a care plan in case something happens to me. As Linda's disease progresses, I will become less mobile. When that happens I will learn to play the piano, learn a new language, and write a book, but for now I am learning to be a better cook, meal planner, and shopper.

Since retiring, I have been building an airplane with my brother. We are due for a test flight in the spring. I have purchased a piano and have begun an outline for the book I will write for my grandchildren.

Linda and I are closer than we have ever been. We have come together to deal with a problem that affects both of us. There are things we wanted to do together that are no longer realistic. But these things are wants and not needs. Relationships and learning count. These are needs that last into eternity. Our strong spiritual underpinnings give us encouragement, strength, and perspective as this Alzheimer's journey continues.

One evening, Linda sat down next to me and said, "I miss the great conversations we used to have. I miss the person I used to be." All we could do was hug each other and shed a few tears. If I had the power to change our lives, I would choose to have Linda be well because she is the best and most refined and valuable part of who we are as a couple.

8

It Has to Be Enough

STEPHANIE STAMM

My sister Carol is twenty years older than I am and has been a sort of second parent as well as a sister to me. When I was less than a year away from completing the requirements for my graduate degree, I accepted her offer to move in with her and her long-time partner, Marilyn.

I ended up living with them for two years while I finished my dissertation and looked for a full-time position. After finding work locally as a technical writer, I moved into a small rental house they owned across the street from their home, renting for a year or so before buying it from them. I had been living first with and then near Carol and Marilyn for five years when my sister was diagnosed with younger-onset Alzheimer's. She was fifty-seven years old.

Carol had retired a couple of years before—a year after Marilyn had done so—and they had planned on a long retirement spent traveling in their motor home. They were only about a year into that plan when it became clear that something was wrong with Carol.

Both Carol and Marilyn had been very successful academics: Marilyn, a dean and then vice president at a liberal arts college; Carol, a professor and then an associate vice president at a state university. As a professor, Carol had taught statistics. Now, she found she couldn't make the correct change when buying small items at the grocery store. And she was, as she described it, "losing words."

Marilyn began handling more of the financial transactions and covering for Carol's slips in conversation when out with friends. They also began the seemingly endless cycle of medical tests, waiting for results, followed by more tests and more waiting. Finally, after another year, when all other possibilities had been eliminated, they received the diagnosis that forced them to relinquish any hopes of recovery.

Marilyn began in earnest to take on the role of caregiver for her life-partner. They still managed to travel, spending the winter after Carol's diagnosis at their favorite campground in Louisiana. But as time passed, Carol's abilities continued to decline, and more and more responsibilities fell to Marilyn.

Then the unthinkable happened. Just before Thanksgiving in 2003, Marilyn started experiencing pain and nausea. She assumed it was just a virus, but when she felt no better the week after Thanksgiving, she finally went to the doctor. She was stunned to learn that she had colon cancer.

All resources were now directed toward Marilyn's recovery. She had to defeat the cancer because she had to take care of Carol. As Marilyn underwent her first rounds of chemotherapy, friends and family stepped forward to help—driving Marilyn and Carol to their respective doctor's appointments, making meals or giving money to have meals catered, cleaning the house.

I, unfortunately, was commuting to Terre Haute, Indiana, weekly for work—a five-hour drive each way. The assignment had started in October. I'd leave early Monday morning and usually get back late Thursday night or early Friday. Sometimes, I'd arrive to find a message telling me Marilyn was in the hospital.

It was during her first hospital stay that Marilyn finally began to refer to Carol openly as her "partner." They had been intensely closeted over the years—largely because of their academic careers but also because both were very private people. They had only told *me* a few months before I moved in with them—by which time they had been together for almost twenty years—and that was because I asked.

We were in their motor home, going I-can't-remember-where for a "camping" trip, and I finally just asked the question. After some moments of shocked silence, they laughed, a little uncomfortably, and answered in the affirmative, acknowledging that they had known they would have to tell me soon, anyway. "Now that you know," Marilyn commented, "you'll be surprised to find that little will change in how we act around you."

In the face of Carol's Alzheimer's and Marilyn's cancer, however, the need for secrecy disappeared. Marilyn wanted to be sure that the hospital staff knew Carol was her life-partner and should be accorded the privileges of family. As soon as she was able, she also contacted their lawyer, and they redid their wills, assigning durable power of attorney for Carol to one of their closest friends and making arrangements for Carol to be financially cared for in the event of Marilyn's death.

Marilyn battled her cancer for thirteen months. During some of this time, she rallied. The chemo was working; the cancer cells were retreating. She felt good, and she and Carol managed another motor-home vacation. Then her condition once again took a downturn. The chemo stopped working; the cancer was growing again.

For four of those months, until I could get myself transferred to a different project that would allow me to be home during the week, I spent my weeks in Terre Haute and much of my weekends with my sister and Marilyn—especially after an act of carelessness on my part forced me out of the denial stage of the grieving process.

During one of the weekends when Marilyn was in the hospital, I'd promised to pick Carol up from there and take her home for dinner. I had plans with a friend earlier in the day and ended up leaving my friend's house later than expected, so I arrived at the hospital later than Carol's usual dinner time. Marilyn soundly berated me, stating that she'd already called a friend to come and get Carol since I hadn't shown up.

It wasn't as if Carol could just go to the hospital snack bar and get something to eat—she couldn't find her way there and back. I hadn't let myself realize that my sister's condition was that bad; what I had viewed as being "a little late" was incredibly disruptive for her—and distressing for Marilyn, who, even from the hospital bed, was trying to protect and take care of her.

Each weekend, in addition to visiting, helping with meals, and portioning Carol's and Marilyn's medicines for the week into their respective weekly pill containers, I'd take Carol on an outing of some sort. We might go out for lunch, go anti-quing, get her haircut, or go shopping for something she needed.

One day, we went shopping for walking shoes. Our visit to the shoe store was rather lengthy, the simple process of trying on shoes having become quite difficult for Carol. She had trouble keeping track of which foot had a shoe on and which did not. I'd touch the socked foot to indicate that it was the one to lift so I could help put a shoe on it. Sometimes the touch helped, but sometimes she lifted the other foot. It had taken a while to find a pair of shoes.

Afterward, we went to one of Carol's favorite lunch spots for Coney dogs. While we were waiting for our food, she looked at me and said, "I try not to be a mess, but I can't help it."

"Oh, honey, I know," I said, reaching to take her hand, my eyes filling with tears.

Marilyn died in January of 2005, making it through one last Christmas. She and Carol had always loved Christmas, filling the house with decorations and piling presents under the tree. I did the shopping for both of them that year. Carol came with me sometimes, but Marilyn was only going out for doctor's appointments by then. Both our families came to Michigan to spend the holidays with Carol and Marilyn. We did it big that year.

Friends and family are convinced that Marilyn lasted as long as she did because of Carol. She fought to stay with her and to spend that last holiday with her.

Carol's condition somehow improved on the day of Marilyn's memorial service. Although, she needed help as usual with things, like picking out clothes and getting dressed, she was more like her old self with people. She talked more, interacted more smoothly—as if willing herself to be as fully present as possible for this final tribute to the love of her life.

Afterward, she seemed to decline more rapidly. Without Marilyn to care for her, she could no longer live in their home. After a month with a live-in caregiver during the week and a friend and me alternating weekends, we moved Carol to Kentucky to live with my brother and his wife, who lived next door to our mother. Carol lived with them for about eighteen months, by which time her condition had deteriorated enough that they could no longer care for her.

In late 2006, we moved Carol to an assisted living facility. We chose one in Kalamazoo, Michigan, since that's where she had lived with Marilyn and where she had her largest circle of friends.

It has been seven years since Marilyn's death. My sister has lost almost everything: her home, her partner, her speech, herself. She is in a different assisted living facility now. We moved her after a few years because she needed more care than the first facility could provide. They suggested a nursing home, but we found another assisted living facility where they have more staff and more care options. They will be able to care for her until the end, involving hospice when that time comes.

I visit my sister. I make sure she has toiletries and clothes. I bring her cake on her birthday. Sometimes she smiles at me. I no longer know if she knows I'm her sister, if she recognizes my face as somehow familiar, or if she's just smiling because she sees a face, any face at all. I talk to her, but she doesn't usually respond. If she does, it isn't in words that I recognize.

As no doubt do most of us who have lost someone dear to Alzheimer's, I too feel incapacitated by the disease. I am helpless to help my sister in any way that feels as if it matters. I can't take away her disease by changing her clothes. I can't take away my grief by feeding her. I can't make her see me as she used to see me by showing up to visit her every week. All I can do is ensure she has a place to stay where she is well cared for, make sure she has the clothes and toiletries that she needs, and visit. It seems so little, but it has to be enough.

9

The Two of Us

PEGGY MITCHELL

My mother was born in June of 1929, one of five children born into an interracial marriage and raised as a black child in Springfield, Illinois. Her parents were in love, devoted to each other until the end. Granddad worked as a cook for the executives of a railroad. He worked extra as a server for parties and exclusive white-only clubs. My grandmother never worked outside her home. He worked, and she saved.

Because of her white ethnicity, Grandmother could buy property all over town. Although they owned rental property around the city, my grandparents lived in a large home in the colored section of town. Mom grew up feeling privileged. Her parents owned cars, a beautiful home and traveled the country through the railroad for free.

My mother always had a job since she was fourteen years old. She worked as an upstairs maid, a basket girl at the lake beach house, and a waitress at a country club. After high school, she was hired by Illinois Bell as the first black telephone operator. She grew up and married a good-looking, smooth-talking man from the wrong side of town without her parents' permission.

They eloped and notified their parents months later. Granddad and Grandmother's reaction was, "You made your bed; now lie in it." Her family knew him because it was a small community, but he was not raised the same way. No one ever imagined she would become his wife. He was not seen as good enough for her.

My mother and father went on to have four daughters beginning in 1951, then 1956, then 1957, and the last in 1961. We were raised as black women, strong and proud of our heritage. All my sisters are married with children. My mother had breast cancer at thirty-five years old and then again at seventy. Her oldest daughter, my sister Billie, also had breast cancer and died at age forty in 1995.

My father passed in 2001. My mother was left alone in our family home. Our journey with health changes began in 2004. My mother first had a heart attack. She recovered very well, attended cardiac rehabilitation, and even drove herself daily. Things seemed to be going fairly well when my mother confided to me that she was having a difficult time paying her bills on time.

She asked me to take over paying her monthly bills. We had the sense to realize it was time to draw up a will and power of attorney in case her health continued to deteriorate. Calls also began to come to me in a St. Louis suburb one hundred miles away from Mom's neighbors. One said, "Your mom's tractor broke down, and she pushed it up a hill alone at seventy-five years old." Another caller said, "Your mom is arguing with us about a road that has been going across her property for over twenty years." And more came. "Your mother went out at seven in the morning for some milk. She lost control of her car, hit a curb, and busted her tire." There was no reason for her to go out so early. It was events like these that would have me speeding down the highway to put out fires and repair damages.

My husband and I had a family meeting and came up with a plan to build an addition to our home for my mother to live in. She could attend activities our children were involved in. We could eat meals together, instead of her eating alone every night. She would not have a three-acre yard to keep up, I could monitor her health care, and she would never need a nursing home. I am a licensed nurse practitioner and felt as though whatever health care issues she had I would be able to handle at home. After all, I had been in home health care for more than thirty years.

So we began our journey. We came up with a house plan, broke ground, and built a handicap-accessible living room, bathroom, and bedroom. At the same time, we began the difficult task of dismantling the home my parents had lived in for more than fifty years and putting it up for sale one hundred miles away. During this period, my mother had a mini-stroke while visiting us one weekend. Her memory seemed to decline again. She could not remember the events of the weekend.

Then the big moving day in December 2008 arrived, My youngest sister, who had also lived in our hometown, moved five miles away from me and came that same day to help with Mom's care. We got all moved in and unpacked boxes. At first we drove Mom everywhere because she had only visited and was unfamiliar with the surrounding area. She had never lived in such a large area, and we were concerned about her safety. She was now having a difficult time remembering how to use her cell phone.

She could answer it but not dial it. She was able to drive to my younger sister's home five miles down the same street. When asked how to get somewhere, she gave wrong directions most of the time, which meant we had to drive her more frequently. She left pots and pans cooking on the stove until they were boiling or burning. We had to make sure she did not prepare snacks that required cooking for her or our children. We began to leave notes and paper for her to write down messages. We put up a list of family members' phone numbers, as well as our own and our address, which she was unable to remember.

Mom soon began to change, not only physically but also mentally. If we left the house, we left her a note saying where every person was and who would be back first. She began to teeter between realizing she needed help to fighting us about her independence. She started to walk away from home in anger with her wallet and money. It would take my sister coming home from work and picking her up or my husband using threats of police intervention to get her to come back home.

We sought help from her primary care doctor who sent us to a neurologist. The neurologist was close to her age and seemed to sympathize with the lack of independence we gave her. I asked him, "What is my mother's diagnosis?" He replied, "She's getting older, just some dementia. We will all experience it if we live long enough." He gave no suggestions where to turn for support. I asked him one day about the Alzheimer's Association. His reply was, "Sure, they are good at what they do. Call them if you want." He prescribed a medicine to slow down her memory loss. The first medication was a patch, which gave her a rash. So we gave her the tablet form, but that led to diarrhea. He changed it to a different medication, and she did seem to stabilize.

Two years later, I began working part-time three days a week. My husband was working fifty miles from home, and my oldest son was attending college away from home. My mother was angry. My youngest son has Down's syndrome. He has daily door-to-door van service, so someone had to be home to receive him, according to school rules. Fortunately, the bus driver had our home phone number and called our house frequently to alert my mom that the van had arrived.

As a family, we agreed to share responsibilities for caring for my mother. Still, Mom often took matters into her own hands. For example, she decided to move into a senior assisted living community. There was no way she could afford this or safely live alone. So we took her to see her neurologist. To quell Mom's anger, I let my sister accompany her to the neurologist. They came out with a note on the prescription pad that read, "Call social services at a hospital to evaluate for assisted living."

The neurologist had recommended this course of action. I tried to explain to her and Mom that social services were for patients in the hospital only, but they didn't believe me. So I called social services and put them on speakerphone. The lady who answered explained they only assisted with hospitalized patients and only those who had no family to help them find financial assistance.

Mom returned home with me, and her anger seemed to dissipate over the next few days. We left her alone. She seemed to forget about the events of the previous week, and her mood improved. During this time, I contacted the Alzheimer's Association. They suggested that Mom see a gerontologist. Mommy, sister, and I went and received good advice on how to manage Mom's anger issues and confusion. The gerontologist advised us to ignore her anger and distract her attention. I should have known this, but we tend to forget good advice when we are in the midst of crisis. Our family practitioner prescribed some different medication, and that helped as well.

Mom no longer likes to cook, but she still wipes out the kitchen sink several times a day. She sweeps the laminate in big sweeping motions that send dust flying everywhere. We learned not to put a glass in the sink or set it on the counter because she will see it and rush in to wash anything left over two minutes. Her dirty laundry has to be folded before going into the hamper. Her white clothes are stacked on the left side of the hamper and darks on the right.

Many of her clothes are in dry cleaning bags and garment bags. She saves every plastic bag available. She hides them in several places around the house. She no longer remembers how to manage her financial affairs. She loves to shop and buy things, not only for herself but also for everyone. It is difficult to keep her on task when she is shopping. She sees something for everyone but herself and gets angry if redirected. Mom has always been generous and put us before herself, but this is so different. Then she tells everyone how I won't let her spend her own money she worked so hard to earn for more than fifty years. Some people understand, but others do not realize the scope of her illness and give me funny looks.

I was diagnosed with breast cancer in June of 2011 and received chemotherapy for two months as the first treatment. I had a bilateral mastectomy in November of 2011. Mom had a stroke in January of 2012 as I was beginning the six weeks of radiation. She and I recovered nicely. It left her with left-sided weakness. I had a minor burn. We both have been going to physical therapy together a few blocks from home. This week Mom fell in her closet, a beautiful closet with a sky light and lots of shelves. She fractured her hip.

Now where will this road lead us, the two of us?

10

Forgetting My Lines

KATHLEEN O'CONNOR

When I started my professional career, I worked in the provost's office at the University of Washington. One of the vice provosts returned from a retreat and regaled us with the following story:

There was a young man who was in his first play. He was to be a page in the king's court. He had only one line: "Hark, the cannon!" A loud explosion off stage would be the cue to say his line. The cast rehearsed and rehearsed, but firing a cannon was difficult and expensive, so they just banged some pans together, and he said his line, "Hark, the cannon!"

They went into dress rehearsal and found a big drum to be the cannon, and he said his line, "Hark, the cannon!" Finally the big night came, and the audience filled the theater. The young man was giddy with excitement. All was going very well, and then the real cannon's sound exploded through the theater. The young man turned quickly and said, "What the hell was that?"

Which is exactly how I felt when I became my mother's caregiver.

As a professional, I worked in health care, largely as a marketing communications and consumer advocate. I specialized in taking complex health care information and putting it into language consumers could understand. I also worked in health care reform working on issues ranging from health care policy to access to health care services. In short, I knew health care like the palm of my hand.

I also knew the science of Alzheimer's disease as it existed then. I was familiar with the range of behaviors and available community resources. I was as prepared as anyone could be for my mother's diagnosis.

Until the cannon of my mother's behaviors exploded.

My father died suddenly of a heart attack in April 1999. I am an only child. My parents lived in San Diego, while I lived in Seattle—a two-and-a-half-hour flight away. I packed and ran out the door to the airport.

As a child, one expects parents to be the decision makers or at least to make their own good decisions. I had not been home since my mother had had a stroke about a year before. We came from a family that never talked about anything medical, as my father had been raised as a Christian Scientist.

I began noticing changes in my mother right away. I noticed she no longer drank alcohol and that she had difficulty finding the right words. My mother could not complete her crossword puzzles. Instead, she cut them out every day and put them in a Japanese letterbox. She did not know how to work the remote control to turn on the television. She did exactly the same thing each day—get up, turn on the stereo, and play the same CDs. We tried to discuss my father's funeral, but she was overwhelmed. To me that was a sign that she was still in shock at my father's sudden death.

I soon realized, however, that it was more than shock. I started going to San Diego, eventually at least once a month, to deal with a multitude of issues. I was facing incredible pressure from my mother's friends—"Whatever you do, don't take her from this house. She loves this house."

It seemed to me at the time that my mother was manufacturing problems so I would have to come back to San Diego. Having lost a son, I understood the grieving process and knew that she would be in shock after my father's death, but I assumed she would get through her grief with her network of friends and some devoted neighbors.

But she was doing things that did not make sense. Even with my professional background, I could not figure out the true cause of her behavior. She no longer knew the difference between a real check and a frequent flyer mileage coupon. She would undercook the chicken in the microwave. She would leave food out for days. When we went out to a restaurant, I was terrified when I had to go to the restroom—wondering if she would still be there when I returned.

I slowly grew aware that my mother should not be living alone. Her neighbors were supportive of that decision. They told me stories of what they were doing for her, about her "broken" remote that her neighbor's husband came once a day to "fix." Her neighbors became her de facto caregivers.

She no longer drove. But when I arrived one time and got to the mail before she did, I found a replacement driver's license. It dawned on me—she was developing crafty behaviors.

Intellectually I knew that Alzheimer's patients often have lucid periods when they seem to return to their normal habits. My mother badly wanted to drive again and called the Department of Motor Vehicles to ask for a replacement of her lost driver's license.

At home in Seattle, I dreaded every time the phone rang. Whenever it did, I worried. Once it was the bank asking me if I knew my mother was cashing a check for four hundred dollars once a week and walking home alone.

In spite of all my years in the health care arena, I was not prepared for the emotional toll this all took. I knew instinctively what was going on, but I was not prepared for the physical impact of dealing with my mother and her health. I knew all about respite care for caregivers. Yet I did not expect the lump in my stomach as I sorted the mail with my mother or helped her in the kitchen. I knew caregivers became exhausted. But I had no idea that the exhaustion is both physical and emotional from walking on egg shells all the time wondering what the next situation would be.

I hired someone in San Diego to visit my mother and check on her periodically, but it was clear that she could no longer live by herself. Because she made little sense talking with people, her friends stopped coming by. Both her world and mine had collapsed. Within six months, neighbors, friends, and I were all saying, "She can't stay in her home anymore."

As a health care professional, I knew where to find resources but had no practice evaluating them. Finding a reliable place for my mother became the next daunting task. I tried to keep her in San Diego, but it was too far away with no consistent care. Even she agreed that she should move to Seattle.

My mother was an elegant woman, so I tried to find a place in Seattle that would be pleasing to her. It was a new for-profit retirement community with an Alzheimer's unit where she could remain independent.

When I came to visit her, I usually avoided going to her room. One day when I did, I was stunned. Her apartment was a mess. The toilet and shower were filthy. I didn't know when it had last been vacuumed.

I never would have suspected this disarray. I discovered that my mother and a male resident in the early stages of Alzheimer's disease would spend hours together. If he was in her apartment, they would not clean it. It also turns out that the medical staff did not monitor her medications. For days they neglected to make notations about her medications.

Of course, I had heard all sorts of stories about elder abuse and neglect. I never thought to question whether my own mother's living space would be kept clean or her medications monitored. I moved her out and even got a partial refund.

Overwhelmed by the task of searching for a new place, I hired someone to help me find a good adult family home for my mother, so she would still feel she was in a residential setting. We found her an appropriate home. Unfortunately, a new owner subsequently raised the fees.

Once again, I located a health system that provided residential oversight of adult family homes and offered health care services. My mother was able to live quite happily there and was well loved and cared for. She died there one year later.

I had blithely thought at the beginning that I knew what I was doing because I knew so much about Alzheimer's and health care. I found a vast difference exists between theory and practice. I had the theory down pat. Cannons in my personal Alzheimer's voyage kept exploding around me erasing all the lines I had memorized in my professional life.

11

A Tale of Gratitude

KARL THUNEMANN

Both my parents had Alzheimer's disease. Their problems began in the 1990s after my father had retired and they moved to Santa Rosa, California. They pursued their interest in the out-of-doors, and my father was deeply involved in his volunteer work as a deacon in the Episcopal Church.

My father, Paul Bryant Thunemann, was born in Portland, Oregon, in 1918. He spent most of his career working as a case manager in wholesale credit. My mother, Muriel Beckman Thunemann, was born in Hubbard, Oregon, in 1920. She was a homemaker and a writer. They met on the University of Oregon campus in Eugene and married in 1940. They had three children.

I first became aware that my parents had memory problems during the early 1990s. My mother became increasingly depressed, partly in response to an emotional crisis that left my parents estranged from one of their children. Later she had a transient ischemic attack—a TIA, or mini-stroke—which she and my father kept secret until they inadvertently revealed it to my brother.

Subsequently, when my wife and I visited, we noticed a dramatic change. My mother intended to cook dinner but could not stay focused. She was caught up in a conversational loop that relied on a few gambits: *What time is it? ... I love what you've done with your hair ... I like your shirt.*

At the time, my father did not seem so impaired. He had a bit of aphasia that almost seemed charming, easily overcome by playing a version of 20 Questions. But his problems progressed. He voluntarily gave up driving after he was in an accident. Once he went indoors to take a call when we were sitting on the patio; suddenly I realized he was giving personal information about his bank account to a stranger.

He became obsessed with errors he made while serving as a deacon on Sunday mornings. He thought he should resign, but the priest insisted he continue. I began visiting my parents frequently and getting involved in their lives. Soon their friends told me that they should not be living alone.

Their general practitioner sent my parents for tests and told me she did not think that either of them had Alzheimer's. But all their friends said they weren't thriving, and I persuaded my father that they should come to Washington and move into assisted living. My mother was adamantly opposed to moving.

She insisted she was fine and took offense at anyone who suggested otherwise. My father took on the heroic task of cajoling her into the move. In some ways, this was his finest hour. It almost seemed that he was staving off his own dementia to take care of her. He knew he had problems, but he strove to allow her to be as normal as he was.

Once they had moved, just sitting in on appointments with a new doctor led me to see how poorly both of them did on the Mini Mental Status Exam. My mother could answer virtually none of the questions. My dad's answers were interesting, even though they were rated as inaccurate. He couldn't name the current president (George W.

Bush) but said he had voted for his opponent. This from a lifelong Republican!

The doctor didn't disclose her diagnoses but did prescribe Aricept to both of them. So I deduced that they had Alzheimer's by looking for the drug on the Internet.

I readily shared the diagnosis with family and close friends. But what was I to tell my parents? My father knew about Alzheimer's. Though he openly discussed his deficits, he clearly did not want to discuss what he called the "dreaded disease." I decided not to tell and soon realized it was likely somebody else would. Their new attorney showed my mother a doctor's letter stating that because my mother had mid-stage Alzheimer's she was incompetent to sign changes to their legal papers. My mother raged for five or ten minutes. Then she subsided, and the topic never came up again.

I sought the support and advice of my family, primarily my wife. She did not often see my parents, but she spent hours bolstering me and was great at making arrangements. I also talked frequently with my mother's younger sister and always asked her opinions on major issues. I consulted with my brother, who visited two or three times a month. I kept my sister informed but didn't seek her advice, as she and our parents had been estranged for several years. I found support at the local Episcopal Church, where a younger priest established immediate rapport with my father and allowed him to resume his work as a deacon. They worked together for nearly two years until my dad was too impaired to continue.

My brother and I had one sharp disagreement over whether our parents should be allowed to go walking in the neighborhood surrounding their assisted living facility, which was on a busy street. He thought it was too risky for them. I knew they had always loved to walk and thought that even with all their faculties they would have preferred to die in an activity they loved than to be locked away.

During my first year, I grew terribly depressed. I wasn't providing personal care for my parents, but I visited them several times a week. And no matter what I did for my father, he always wanted more. But at least I was engaged with him. I was not my mother's favorite child, but we had always had a good connection. As her capacity to recognize me diminished, she viewed me with suspicion and sometimes hostility.

I decided to seek a part-time job: I needed the money AND I needed to be less available. By a curious synchronicity, I wound up working as a specialist on the Alzheimer's Association's 24/7 Helpline. I applied after calling the helpline for resources. The job was listed on the chapter's website. It was the only job I applied for.

You might think this would lead to an overdose of dementia, but for four years it was anything but. My new colleagues encouraged me to set limits with my parents. I used my time with them more effectively. Instead of looking on dispiritedly as my parents declined, I could help other people facing similar circumstances. Instead of wondering if I was doomed to dementia myself, being forced to learn this large volume of information in a short time affirmed that my mind remained adept and flexible—and I had a place to use it. My colleagues were very supportive, and I was blessed to be able to work with the association's clients, who repeatedly impressed me with their strength and courage.

My parents stayed in assisted living for two years until my mother had a couple of falls that landed her in a nursing home. She would not be allowed to return. I engaged a housing specialist who found a place that was not far from my dad's church. But he didn't like it. So I expanded the geographical target area and found a place that was nearly perfect. In a short time, my mother bonded with the chief caregiver—and her daughter, who also worked in the home.

Over the next three years, my mother showed a new side—she became girlish, teasing, and playful, a favorite in the home. It was not so easy for my dad, who imagined the chief caregiver had usurped his role of taking care of my mother. He was angry, and there was talk of requiring him to move alone to a locked ward. But the chief caregiver fought doggedly to keep him.

A few weeks after my mother died (there had been several deaths in the home within a few months), the chief caregiver and her daughter were fired—without cause, as far as I could tell. I was extremely angry and gave notice to move my father, though I had no idea where. The fired caregiver offered to take him into her home. And there he lived for the last three years, a treasured member of her large extended family, invited to all family outings (which sometimes were cancelled if he was too ill to travel).

I am still grateful to my parents for choosing me to look after them and was sorry that my siblings didn't have this opportunity. I am especially grateful for the opportunity to grow close to my father during these years after a lifetime of difficulties.

How has caregiving affected me? I can't ascribe any physical change. I'm certainly glad I didn't try to care for them at home. I considered myself to be free of racial, ethnic, and social bias when I came to work for the association. I found that wasn't completely true, so working in that setting was cleansing. Dementia is so much bigger than the miniscule differences that too often divide people. I think most of my biases dissolved.

As for how it has affected me spiritually, it is difficult to assess my own progress. I *think* I am better attuned to accepting mortality, to living in the moment and not being in a hurry. Caregiving has changed many of my ideas about life and death. I no longer think it would be so terrible to die of a heart attack or a stroke, especially if I didn't linger. I try to think of my life as complete. I still have things I want to do, but my ambition has shifted. I try to see these activities more as *process* than projected *product.*

Here are lessons I think might help other caregivers who are just beginning their journey with Alzheimer's. First, if you are an adult child taking care of a parent with dementia, be prepared to revisit all the emotional issues you have had with that parent. On the helpline, I learned that this challenge is virtually inevitable—no matter how much work you have done already on those issues.

Second, if you are an older adult taking care of a spouse at home, get help! I can't begin to estimate how often I talked to gallant old women (and a few men!) who had to do everything, either from love or from a spouse's refusal to accept help. *You can't do everything yourself!* It will put you in an early grave.

Third, if you are caring for a spouse who has early-onset Alzheimer's, go to one of the association's support groups designed to serve you. When I felt at a loss when receiving calls about early onset, I asked to sit in on a group with this focus. These spouses are incredibly honest and open with each other, and they helped me see how I should respond.

Fourth, and finally, whatever form your caregiving takes, do at least one thing a week just for yourself. It's not self-indulgence but essential for mental health.

12

Home, at Last

JEANNE TRIPSANSKY

The director of nursing at my mother's Alzheimer's residential care facility in northern Indiana interrupted me one day in the middle of my work with unsettling news. She informed me that my mother required skilled nursing care at a nursing home or 24/7 assistance from a private caregiver in order to remain at the facility.

At the time, I was working as a hairdresser for residents at the Alzheimer's and assisted living facility where my mother had resided for sixteen months. The director explained that my mother had to move to a different facility because she no longer fulfilled the criteria under the original contract. To say I was startled would be an understatement.

I wondered what criteria she referred to. I later learned that my mother failed to meet all three requirements of state regulations. She was incontinent and could no longer transfer or feed herself.

Already her decline was apparent to me. I had fed her lunch on those days that I worked, bought her adult briefs for several years, and helped her as she transitioned from a walker to a wheelchair three months earlier. Her condition had greatly diminished during the past six months. My mother talked less, had difficulty walking, and lost weight. In early spring, I began receiving more calls about her falls.

She didn't suffer any serious bumps or fractures, and her vital signs were normal, but no one ever saw her fall. My mother sometimes fell out of bed or fell in the hallway. Each fall meant she needed additional care. Nurses installed bed rails, gave her a walker and eventually a wheelchair, and provided occupational therapy. The progression of events was predictable, but watching her decline was excruciating. Alzheimer's stripped her of her identity and the ability to care for herself. What a cruel disease.

I left work that day stunned, scared, angry, anxious, and overwhelmed. I had believed Mom would not have to move again, except to the funeral home. I always anticipated the call that she had passed. I was troubled to learn for the fifth time in eight years that she had to leave the facility as soon as possible. On my drive home, I stopped to meet the director of the Alzheimer's services hoping to quell the growing panic inside me. She provided me with a list of residential facilities, private residential homes, and in-home care options. Mainly, she helped me accept the reality of my mother's situation and reduce my fear and anxiety. The truth was that Mom had late-stage Alzheimer's disease.

After many years of wondering, asking, pleading, and praying for her to be released from this horrific condition, the time of decision was at hand. As I continued my drive home, I decided to visit a senior community center with skilled nursing located twenty minutes from my home, which was more convenient than my current forty-minute drive. I was staggered to learn that it would cost $7,000 per month, private pay. Mom's money would be gone in less than a year.

Mom's long-term-care insurance expired at the beginning of the year, and she was not eligible for Medicaid. What's more, many of the care facilities did not accept Medicaid. Her current rent of $4,300 was manageable, but $7,000 was not. I drove home weighing the options. I ruled out a nursing home facility. A private residential home was still an option. Hiring someone to come to our home to provide extra help was another. We had tried keeping her in our home five years earlier when we had to find a place immediately after being told the facility would not be liable for her.

Caring for my mother was the last thing I ever thought I would do. Our relationship was cordial, without affection. We were not close, nor did we confide our personal selves. I thought of her as the Ice Queen—cold, uninvolved, and critical—and believed she didn't like me.

After my father's passing, she was no longer able to manage her day-to-day life and needed someone else to be in charge. My older brother, and only sibling, lived close to her but was too busy to be involved. I was resentful. I worked full-time as an environmental scientist; I wasn't ready to give up my career. And how would my husband of two years feel about this? I felt fear, anxiety, coupled with dread of what was to come. And, what was to come?

Caring for Mom in our house was the best option. In addition, our rural home had a fenced yard. We painted and carpeted the downstairs bedroom, installed secured locks on doors. We genuinely believed that keeping her at home would work. I made a decision to leave my job, without notice, in order to care for her at home.

The first week was a breeze, but then Mom became delusional. She began imagining that someone was breaking in. Evenings were the worst. She was overcome by fear and anxiety and knocked over furniture crying for help. We were exhausted and losing our minds too. I called her doctor seeking help; he arranged to hospitalize my mother for seventy-two hours, enough time for me to find another housing solution. On that last day in our home, she was calm and congenial. We sat together that day working on a jigsaw puzzle. She talked about how she enjoyed being at her high school class reunion and spoke as if I was one of her fellow classmates. She had no idea of who I was or where we were.

From the start of this ten-year journey when I became my mother's primary caregiver, my husband and I agreed that we would bring her home to spend her final days. When the time finally arrived, my husband never wavered. "Of course she comes here," he said. We had plenty of room, so we began planning for her return. This time would be different. We asked the hospice team and the visiting physician to continue their service. We also hired additional daytime help.

We could do this. On August 31, 2011, I went to work at mom's Alzheimer's unit. I completed my hairdresser appointments by noon. While Mom was in the dining room, I finished emptying her room of clothing, pictures, and toiletries. Within a short time, her room was empty, and my car's trunk and back seat were full. I asked one of the nursing aides, a young woman with great compassion for her clients, to help me transfer Mom into my car. We wheeled Mom out of the lock-down facility into the warm, sunny afternoon light.

The aide grasped Mom under the arms lifting her up and out of the wheelchair, forcing her to stand up. "What are you doing?" my mother exclaimed. The aide steadied her on her feet, slowly turned her around, and guided her to the front car seat. Once Mom was settled, head hanging down, eyes closed, quiet, and we were alone in the car, I told her that she was coming home. How many times had she asked, "Don't I have a home to go to?" or said, "Mom's waiting for me; I want to go home."

The forty-five-minute drive was quiet and reflective. My mind traced back over the ten years since my father's death and this Alzheimer's journey began. He tried to tell me that Mom's memory was failing but never told me the whole truth. She had been diagnosed with vascular dementia two years prior to my father's passing, a fact I learned five years after his death. I did the best I could. In the earlier stages, she would ask, "What's going to happen to me?"

I always responded that we would keep her safe, protect and provide for her. She insisted that she did not want to live with us. She remembered her own grandmother living with her family and the frightening memories of her father restraining his mother. One of Mom's sisters also suffered with Alzheimer's. Yet, here we were, the last time in my life that I would travel this quiet rural countryside with my mother.

In the process of caring for my mother, many old wounds healed. We became friends; we said, "I love you." Early on, she acknowledged that she trusted me and was thankful that I returned home and cared for her. Our roles changed; I was parenting my parent. Within a few years, she stopped call me by my name, Jeanne; instead, she called me Phyllis, a childhood friend. She often asked if she and I were related, was I her mother or sister? She told me I was her favorite lady.

I knew that our mission from now on was to help her die, and I prayed that it would be peaceful, calm, and filled with love, joy, and compassion.

My husband was waiting when I drove through the front gate. When he helped turn and lift her up out of the car, she yelled again, "What are you doing?" It took both of us to support her as she tried to walk into the house, across the living room, and into the room we had prepared for her. She was dead weight, unable to stand on her own. I didn't know she was this incapable of walking. The facilities staff said that she was able to stand and walk with little assistance, maybe for them but not for us. We managed to get her into the hospital bed that the hospice workers had arranged for delivery the day before.

The hospice nurse soon arrived and helped to undress Mom from a worn-out sweat suit into a fresh hospital gown. Mom was strong and fought with her arms, grabbing whatever she could get hold of, and complained loudly. Once she was clean, changed, and settled, I saw her reach out and grasp the bed rail. For a moment, she appeared to have a look of fear, and then acceptance settled in. She was safe at home. Mom passed away peacefully, gently, and quietly seventeen days after coming home. I learned to love her in a way I never had before. It was an honor to care for her and experience her death with love, joy, and compassion.

Part Three

Portraits in Compassion

Love and compassion are necessities, not luxuries.
Without them, humanity cannot survive.

- His Holiness, the Dalai Lama

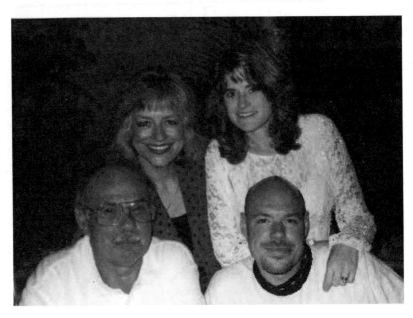

The Tatalias Family

13

George's Story

BABS TATALIAS

L ife takes strange turns. Never could I have imagined that
I'd help the man whom I had divorced two decades ago. I
will forever remember that sinking feeling when our daughter
called with the awful news of George's diagnosis of early-onset
Alzheimer's. I feel it right now.

I had read enough about this disease to know this was
just about as bad as news can get. Our grown children, Stefanie
and Todd, had plenty to do with jobs and small children. Even
though I was working full time—and blissfully single—I felt
compelled to help George. I couldn't ignore the man with whom
I had shared so much of my young life, the man with whom I'd
watched the world change. So, more than two decades after our
divorce and a subsequent second, sixteen-year marriage and
divorce for George, I didn't think twice about helping to make
sure that George would be cared for.

One of my first calls was to the Alzheimer's Association
Helpline. Their calm and soothing advice allowed me to hope
that I could meet this challenge. I'll never find adequate words
to express my gratitude to the association.

As a family, we sprang into action. I found a condominium for George in the same Seattle complex where I lived. I worked full time with crazy hours, but I helped George out when I wasn't at work. Our son, Todd, who lived in Alaska, flew to Palm Springs to supervise the sale of George's condo and his move to Seattle. Our daughter, Stefanie, also moved to Seattle.

George at age sixty was so different from the George I had met in 1963. Back then, George was an imposing figure— tall, slender, dark hair, dark suit, and all business. Still, on our first date, he charmed me by his humor, as well as his snazzy Corvette. He was the golden boy of his extended family, the first to go to college and the first to leave his coal-mining hometown. After we married, he successfully climbed the corporate ladder, going from restaurant manager to vice president of a nationwide company.

After our divorce, we didn't talk to each other. His friends said that he never recovered from being let go after twenty years of loyalty.

Before his diagnosis in 1998, during a trip to Chicago for our son's wedding reception, I had learned from George that his second marriage was ending. I was shocked. I thought everything was going well in his life. He lived in one of the most recognizable high rises of the Chicago skyline, with a view that knocked my socks off. He seemed devastated at the turn of events in his life. I felt badly for him. We began talking again.

After his second divorce in 2000, George moved from Chicago to Palm Springs, calling me every night from the road, being friendly, letting me know of his progress. He wasn't quite the George I had known way back then, full of self-confidence and vigor, but he had been through a lot. I didn't think it was more than that.

Our daughter, Stefanie, however, believes that George showed signs of Alzheimer's before he and I reconnected. He covered his forgetfulness and failure to follow through well because not until he lived alone did Stefanie suspect something more serious. She urged him to see a doctor. When he finally did at age sixty, the diagnosis was Alzheimer's.

I began attending a support group for friends and family of early-onset patients sponsored by the Alzheimer's Association. Once George moved to Seattle, we planned to have him live in his own condo. Everyone advised us to rent an apartment. We went ahead and bought one, and luckily, it worked. We also straightened out George's finances, which had been in shambles with large credit card charges. We paid off as many of his debts as we could. George was then able to live alone for more than two years.

His living alone did cause us anxiety. In retrospect, we were truly lucky. We organized things to minimize risk and watched carefully for signs of change. Stefanie prepared meals for him and placed them in individual containers for easy microwaving. For his safety, we unplugged the electric range. It was an easy walk from George's condo to mine. On the evenings I did not work, he came to my place with his containers of food.

When the time came for him to give up his beloved sports car, I worried it would be difficult, but he easily accepted that driving was hazardous to himself and others. Perhaps George was actually scared to drive.

I had volunteered for us to be part of a study sponsored by the University of Washington. At the end of the two-year study, George's precipitous decline was unmistakable. Still, everybody liked him. He had not lost his sense of humor. But for me, his decline was heart wrenching.

I'm trying to remember when we recognized that George should not live alone. Was it when even using the microwave seemed hazardous? Two of them broke. Was it when he called over and over not remembering having called before? Was it the awful thought of George walking out of his home and getting lost?

Just when we needed it, a spot opened up at one of the care facilities recommended by my support group. Stefanie and I had visited other larger facilities. We had also looked at some expensive, privately run group homes. With only twelve residents, the place we chose seemed less institutional. Each of the residents had a small room in a two-story home that looked like any other house on the block. The facility was subsidized for low-income individuals, most of them needing memory care.

I can't say enough nice things about this facility. The mostly North African staff of women was, without exception, warm and caring. The manager took George to the weekly farmer's market nearby when he could still walk. All the cooking was done in the warm kitchen atmosphere, right next to where the residents sat at a large wooden table. Cooking smells wafted through the air; you could almost pretend it was home.

Over the years, much of my caregiving for George went smoothly. I also lived through many "worst moments."

There was the time the doctor from the University of Washington study helped us tell George that it wasn't safe to live alone anymore. We then visited the home he eventually moved to. He didn't want to go inside. I remember the look on his face: don't do this to me. It was awful.

Another time, I took George to a neurologist after he moved to Seattle. The doctor asked him to draw the face of a clock. The numbers, one through twelve, wound up all scrunched together on the right side of a circle.

Then there was the day, while driving, that I sang,

Georgie Porgie, pudding and pie,
Kissed the girls and made them cry.

George totally shocked me by wailing like a small child. It was heartbreaking. What memories had I just stirred up?

Possibly the worst time was the day I saw a tear rolling

down George's cheek. He was in his wheelchair, no longer able to walk, talk, or feed himself. My heart sank. I was hoping that, though I had bundled him in warm clothing and wrapped a blanket around him before our walk through the sunny autumn afternoon, the chill air had caused the tear. But I didn't know. Was George aware of what was happening to him? Was that the cause of his tears? The worst part was not knowing what he was aware of or what he needed. Was he warm enough? Were his anti-depressants helping or hurting? Could I do anything more to make him comfortable? Could I do anything more at all?

Fortunately, I remember some good times, too. Before George was wheelchair-bound, I used to take him for mini-road trips. I always had music on, mostly oldies from the fifties and sixties. I would ask him who the recording artist was, and whenever he couldn't come up with the name of the female vocalist, he'd say Patti Page and then laugh, knowing it was a crazy guess.

One of our favorite pastimes was sauntering through the botanical garden with our granddaughter. It was so sweet. George noticed every small pretty flower. During our marriage, he'd never stopped to smell the roses.

The average length of time between diagnosis of early-onset and death is seven years. George passed away just before Christmas 2009, a few months after the seventh year since his diagnosis.

Sometimes I feel good about everything I did. Sometimes I wish I had done more. I'm asked sometimes why I helped at all—we had divorced ages ago. It never occurred to me not to help. We had children together; we had always been a family in that sense. And if I hadn't been there, my children would have had to do it all alone. Todd and Stefanie both had families and small children who needed them. So we all did what was right. End of story.

Over two years after George's death, I still get phone calls and mail for George. On the outside of one envelope from *Golf Digest* imploring him to renew his subscription were these printed words: Come Back, We Miss You.

They have no idea.

14

The Butterfly Effect

STEFANIE TATALIAS

A proverbial phone call changed everything, a call that prompted my sixty-year-old dad and me to move from opposite ends of America when I was thirty-four to face a disease with an inevitably ugly ending.

My dad and I had always been close, even when I ventured around the world. He always applauded my courage and never judged my lifestyle. Although I often traveled solo, helping him as he died of Alzheimer's disease was a far lonelier experience. My friends couldn't relate to my circumstances, and neither did his friends, who seldom called.

Yet, I wasn't alone. Help came from the strangest place, from the woman who had divorced my dad twenty years ago. My mom.

Mom had no reason to step up to the challenge of caregiving. She reached out to both my dad and me. Before this new predicament, my mom seldom seemed to understand my bold decisions or way of speaking. So we often clashed. Yet she was there for me now, without hesitation, complaints, or guilt.

While my friends and colleagues were clueless about Alzheimer's disease, my mom enabled me to become a caregiver, maintain a normal life, and yet not bite people's heads off when they asked, "Does he still remember you?"

If my biggest worry were whether my dad would remember me, it would have been easy. What about whether he'd recall how to turn on the lights, turn off the water, or even form words?

The week before that pivotal phone call, my mom and I had been in Seattle hunting for a condo for Dad. Recently divorced, he wanted to relocate. He wasn't doing well. Worried about whether he had succumbed to drinking or depression, I urged him to see a doctor. The symptoms of memory loss had been creeping up on my sixty-year-old dad for four or five years. He had yet to be diagnosed with Alzheimer's, even after an attempted suicide.

Initially, my mom stipulated that his new place be at least fifteen minutes away from her home. That was before he was diagnosed with Alzheimer's.

Having moved my dad to Seattle, suitcase in hand, I was about to leave Mom's home. Her phone rang. My four- and six-year-old kids were already in the taxi waiting to depart for the airport, the meter and their internal time bombs ticking. I almost ignored the phone, but intuition beckoned. It was my dad's neurologist asking to speak to me. I'm thankful I received the bad news instead of my mom. After his Alzheimer's diagnosis, Mom changed her mind and found a condo for Dad just a short walk from her door.

Once I relocated to Seattle, I delivered dinners to him every few days. When my dad began forgetting to eat, Mom would invite him over. His appetite was small and they'd share dinners. Watching Dad decline tore my mother's heart up, but she relished his company and, I think, the opportunity to dissolve hard feelings left from the divorce.

My own pragmatism helped me in caregiving. When Dad forgot how to dial a phone, I found one with pictures. To quell his angry and sometimes violent behavior, I found a doctor who prescribed anti-psychotic medication. However embarrassing and difficult it was for him, I discovered ways to talk with him about his disease.

I also searched for silver linings. As Dad grew younger in his disposition, my own daughter grew older, so when she was four, they became peers.

Spotting a flowering cherry tree, Dad would say, "Pinky trees!" And Jade would chant, "Mine, mine, and mine."

They'd both laugh. And I'd force myself to find it funny, too, not tragic.

My son, Jevon, felt cheated, however. He would never know the grandfather who once ran the entire food service for Boeing. Jevon did learn to make Dad's favorite Caesar salad.

When my dad moved to an assisted living facility, I visited him almost daily for six months and listened to him say again and again, "They shoot horses, don't they?"

Eventually, he stammered too much to make any sense. Yet, he still seemed to understand us. My boyfriend and I would take him out for dinner or drinks. Guessing at what he was saying, we'd keep the conversation rolling, just to give him a normal experience, away from his declining Alzheimer's housemates.

On his sixty-sixth birthday, Dad was wheelchair-bound and unable to feed himself. Photography had been one of his favorite hobbies, so I bought him a camera. Tearfully, he pressed all the buttons. I hoped they were happy tears.

For me, Dad's Alzheimer's condition brought to life all the spiritual wisdom I'd studied over the years. The Christian virtue of kindness helped me keep giving. Yoga and its emphasis on being gentle and non-harming guided me while making decisions on Dad's behalf. And Buddhism revealed that, though suffering in life is inevitable, we can celebrate the joys of living.

Philosophy aside, without Mom's commitment to caring for Dad, I would have fallen apart. So much was uncertain. Was he in pain? Did he know what was happening to him? My mom and I routinely reassured one another that we, and his caregivers, were doing our best to support him. Working together, my mom and I learned to trust each other.

The butterfly effect tells us that seemingly random and remote actions send out ripples that can bring about momentous change. I propose a corollary: the metamorphosis effect. One person's transformation can directly alter other lives. While caterpillars eventually shed their outward appearance and become butterflies, Alzheimer's patients go in the opposite direction. They appear to grow less beautiful, capable, and human. But I believe when Dad turned inward, he connected with the source of all being.

As my dad withdrew into his cocoon, instead of growing wings for himself, he gave them to me. A heaviness lifted from my heart. I now know just how much my mom loves me. She gave up a huge part of her life to care for her ex-husband … and her daughter. And that has been a priceless gift.

15

From Partner to Parent

VIRGINIA BENSON

Of course I knew of George Benson when I began attending Trinity Church in the summer of 1980 after separating from an impossible marriage. Everyone knew him—his profession as a psychoanalyst gave him a certain cachet, and he was frequently featured in lectures and on television—and his devoted care for his wife, who suffered from brittle diabetes, was very visible. As we became acquainted at various parish events and dinners back and forth, I learned of his wide-ranging interests and accomplishments.

He was a runner and a bicyclist, had traveled extensively, flew an airplane, and was a competent amateur singer and recorder player, among other things. He was handsome and especially dashing in the eighteenth-century-style boatmen's shirts (think Bingham's *Jolly Flatboatmen*) that his daughter had made for him. He was happily married and therefore entirely off-limits, I knew, but I used to wish there were more like him or a way to clone him since my own social life was sadly lacking in interesting straight men.

I went about my business and actually benefitted greatly from those years on my own. I'd been brought up to be a nice girl, to be bright enough to attract the right kind of husband but not be threatening to his superiority, to be amenable and not call undue attention to myself. And the "contract" of my first marriage (I learned that every relationship has a contract, implicit if not overt) reinforced all of that—I was a bit flawed, but he would be tolerant of my deficiencies. Eventually, in my forties, I came to realize that I did not need to be tolerated and, after several years of trying to renegotiate that contract to allow more of a relationship of equals, knew that that would not happen, and if I were to live I needed to get out of the marriage.

I discovered strengths and abilities I'd not realized before (though my friends tell me I was always mouthy and opinionated!) and built a pretty satisfactory life. My volunteer experience led to a modest career in public relations for mostly non-profit organizations. I tried a few jobs that paid better, but my heart wasn't in any of them, and I was able to get work in areas of my passions—the local opera company, the public radio station, the Episcopal diocese. I bought a wonderful small house in a historic district. I had friends and kept busy with a variety of activities. I was lucky enough to have a man friend who presented no romantic possibilities but was a great traveling companion and introduced me to far corners of the world.

Along the way, George invited me to perform with him in a challenging and beautiful Telemann work he had found that he thought would be enjoyable to present at church, with him playing recorder and me doing the vocal part—it also involved a viola da gamba and a harpsichord. Enjoyable it was, and along with some other performances together, we established a bond that might be difficult to understand for people who haven't performed together—it seemed that our souls spoke in unison.

And then, at the end of July 1988, his wife, Anne, died. George and I were already friends, and he had done a lot of his grieving for her during her long illness, and in due course we allowed our friendship (and yes, the bit of attraction that had been there all along) to develop into a love that startled us both with its intensity. We gave it time and worked out the inevitable kinks that any two people have in settling into a relationship. With me, he found a more sociable part of himself, and he helped me find a quiet place within that I had neglected.

The next years were a glorious adventure. A slightly rundown but beautiful and historically significant house called to us and crystallized our awakening desire to make a life together. We had a wonderful wedding with all our aggregate six children involved and many dear friends (it was surprising how many of them were already mutual) helping us to celebrate. The house was demanding but responsive to our efforts, and we had none of the arguments over money, time, or decorating choices that we were told many couples did.

One of St. Louis's early brewers had built the house, and his lively spirit permeated it. George delighted in solving renovation problems, built beautiful bookcases on all three floors, and tended our increasingly elaborate garden. I relished cooking for us and entertaining guests and housing opera singers on our third floor during the season. Our parties were lively—people didn't seem to want to go home. It seemed that George and I had a synergy that created space for our friends to be themselves at their best. At one point early on, George was taking a break from a project, looking around with pleasure at our progress, and thought, "I'm so glad I can do this for her … Wait a minute, I'm not doing it for her; we're doing it *together*." And thus the last vestiges of the Great Doctor's nineteenth century sensibility fell away, and we became a true partnership.

We really didn't register the import of several things that happened during late 2004 and early 2005.

George was feverish one day and that night woke up unsteady, disoriented, and unable to hold his urine. When he fell a second time, I called 911, and we went to the hospital. For three days, he continued to be confused but was diagnosed with a urinary tract infection and treated with antibiotics. The disorientation was not unusual in such a situation, they said, but scheduled a neurological exam. He flunked it flat.

We were flabbergasted at the diagnosis of "probable Alzheimer's." Of course there were things like family finances that he had never wanted to bother with, and actually it was kind of a good thing in his profession that he wasn't very good at remembering names. ("Memory? What memory? He's never had a memory!" said his children when told of it.) So he began a course of one of the standard medications, and some months later, the doctor added the other of the only two that research thought might slow down the progress of the disease. And for quite a while, we could almost forget about it.

We had been observing the progress of development of the old City Hospital into condominiums, and when signs went up announcing the opening of the project, we went to see it out of curiosity. When we emerged from the building, I said, "My piano is prettier than yours, but clearly we can't take both of them into the condo, and yours is a better instrument."

We both knew then that we were ready to give up the big house, and I honestly don't remember if that was before or after he came in from mowing the lawn and said, "This isn't fun anymore." After a period of searching, we found just the right place and eventually sold the house. It was great fun designing the condo just as we wanted it, and we almost laughingly put in grab bars and lever handles so we could live out our days here. We didn't know how lucky we would later feel that we were no longer in a three-story house with a large garden!

George had been fortunate to have his retirement from his practice occur gradually, and during the years in the house, he was occupied with its projects. After we moved and the pictures and the shelves were hung, though, he had little to do since we no longer needed him to do carpentry chores or yard work. He grumbled a bit but realized he now had more time to read and practice the piano, a long-loved but mostly neglected pleasure.

When did the symptoms become intrusive? It's hard to know. Of his own accord, he gave up driving after highway construction made it difficult to make the weekly visits to his colleague and friend who was further advanced in the disease. "My reflexes aren't what they were, and I can't always find my way," he said—and what a boon that was as we realized how many men seem to connect their car keys with a significant part of their male anatomy! Then he began to lose his way returning to our unit from parties in the building. And he had more and more trouble finding the words to express the thoughts that themselves became more elusive.

He cried over hymns at church and over the Honor Roll on the *News Hour*. He would ask, "What does the day look like?" repeatedly each morning and then forget the answer. He spoke more frequently of his parents and his brothers and his youth and most of all the army, and when I would try to prompt a recollection from his adulthood, his professional life, his marriage, raising his children, he would simply go blank. I had kept up with activities and friendships, but he had not, and I realized at some point that he never did maintain associations that were not current. He got anxious when I was away, and if it were an evening thing, he was likely to drink too much.

We connected with the Alzheimer's Association and were much helped by the information, the support group, and the activities they offered. Eventually, though, George could no longer take part in the telephoning of shut-ins or in the support group (he apparently thought he was conducting a therapy group and was harsh with a group member who was having trouble articulating his thoughts). While he still deeply enjoys opera and symphony performances and the cultural excursions to museums and exhibits I try to plan each week, his increasing physical frailty and his tendency to speak aloud during performances makes those more difficult.

Now the most interesting person I have ever known, the love of my life, has the cognitive and emotional capacity of an eight-year-old, according to the "retrogression chart" that Alzheimer's researchers have developed. He's a very bright and personable eight-year-old, to be sure, but he can't be left alone, and he needs help choosing appropriate clothing, and things have to be explained again and again, and I'm forever on the alert to be sure nothing awful happens.

And unlike the eight-year-olds many of us have raised, this bright child will not learn from his experience or benefit from the consequences we carefully insured for our growing offspring. George depends entirely on me, and I'm thankful that he often expresses his love and thanks me for what I do for him. But I didn't expect to be a mother again, and as one support group friend says, I often feel like a single mom.

The marriage that was once a vibrant and synergistic partnership is no more. I can still, sometimes, remember how I simply melted when I looked at him. And from time to time, we share some fun. But I wonder every day how I, or anyone else in my situation, can live a marriage in which one partner is a child.

16

Into the Storm

NANCY GOULD-HILLIARD

We had a roadmap for navigating my husband Bob's Alzheimer's disease, which was diagnosed fourteen years ago when he turned sixty. It was his dad, who suffered memory loss for twenty years, from his mid-sixties to mid-eighties. We watched Pop Hilliard forget his history lectures, lose his independence as a driver after retiring, shadow his wife wherever she went, undergo personality changes, and move into assisted living for his final chapter.

While I had managed Bob's parents' finances and Medicaid paperwork, their journey scarcely prepared me for what would become my emotional walk as Bob's chief advocate. I helped him navigate his final five years as a university professor and student publications' manager as his cognitive curtain began to descend. Together we tackled the medical morass of obtaining diagnosis and treatment plans—and accepted and adapted to each new stage of cognitive loss.

For thirty-two years, Bob has been my ultimate partner since I found him at mid-life. We shared the same passions for journalism, intellectual jousting, devotion to family, gardening, do-it-yourself projects, letter-press type collecting, church, public service, and so many other pursuits. At one time, he had owned a newspaper, worked for major news organizations in California, Idaho, Oregon, and Washington, and spent twenty-two years teaching media relations to the new crop of students. He inspired untold numbers of communicators—including me, who enjoyed his strongest gift as the Great Affirmer that everyone seeks.

As soon as we discovered why Bob was losing his mental acuity, we were determined to make hay while the sun shines. After retiring from our dual university careers, we visited the national parks and our favorite Pacific Northwest retreats ... spent time with grandchildren, families, and friends ... conducted random acts of gardening ... helped feed the homeless ... and grasped as much enjoyment as possible from films, church, and other associations. We even did a marathon walk as we had become daily walkers.

But our bravado slowly began to crumble. On one of Bob's more notorious odysseys, he donned three jackets and quietly slipped out the front door one evening, not to be found until 4 a.m. by the police—fourteen miles from home. That's when we had to put chimes and chain locks on all the doors. I began to recognize that Alzheimer's had all but diminished the old Bob I knew and trusted, and I too became part of the physical lock-down.

We took advantage of the local day-care service for seniors with dementia: Tuesdays and Thursdays at the senior center and several eight-hour shifts a week at an assisted living facility. What a load this took off my daytime plate. We tried in-home companion care, but the expense didn't compensate for the benefits gained. I began attending the local monthly caregivers support group and found a wonderful adult family home a fifteen-minute drive away, which would take Bob for occasional overnights if I needed a getaway.

Sleep became problematic as Bob awoke several times a night. Because of his growing incontinence, it now took more of my energy to assist him with toileting. I also focused on redirecting his delusions, grooming, medicating, and reorganizing both our worlds. Little did I realize the toll this 24/7 caregiving was taking on me until last January when a regular mammogram revealed I had stage-two breast cancer. My doctor firmly told me that I would have to seek other caregiving options for Bob while I focused on my own care for at least six months.

How silly, I thought ... I can take care of the two of us just fine. My own myopia had trumped better judgment. Luckily, a stroke of serendipity arose from the group home I had used for respite care. It had an opening, and Bob began to adjust to his *much* longer stay there.

Home alone for the first time in my life, I sought help from family and friends. They drove me to appointments, accompanied me on my daily one-mile walks, and lifted my spirits in card blitzes and other ways. Four friends began checking up on me daily—and still do. The church brought us home communion—to both the group home and my home. I experienced Reiki, biofeedback, meditation, and physical and counseling therapy as bonuses to the conventional treatments.

We are still, at this juncture, uncertain when our next major adjustment will be necessary. The only certainty is that more changes are inevitable. I grieve for the slow loss of my affirmer and sidekick. My counselors tell me I am over-anxious because of my multiple stresses; but, alas, anxiety medication cannot become my daily helper. I must find other ways to quell my nerves and the deep ache inside me.

I am less cavalier about my ability to be strong at all times, yet I have found new coping mechanisms. At a retreat at the Monastery of St. Gertrude in Cottonwood, Idaho, the nuns taught me self-care: meditation, tai ch'i chuan, the arts as salve, and how to "relax into the tumult, rather than trying to hurry and fix it. Acknowledge it, sit with it a spell, remove its thorn, and give it up to a higher power." How I loved sitting in the nuns' glider chairs and just letting the world turn.

I still deeply miss Bob's companionship. Some days when I visit him, we simply hold each other for five minutes straight. His "salad talk" no longer makes any sense, but his affection remains unmistakable. And then we take our walk, drink in the fresh air, point out the beauties of nature along the way, and return to our separate corners.

A significant stress is the financial burden of Alzheimer's caregiving. It will take its toll in another year or so when the unrelenting costs of monthly care will force me to sell our home for living expenses. We were not able to get long-term care insurance for Bob, even at age sixty, when he was in the early stages. The tests revealed his memory loss even then. He is not a veteran, who can get benefits. And, the nation's health care plan makes no provisions for the 5.5 million who have the disease in America—or their caregivers.

As I watch our retirement fund from careers as educators and journalists dwindle each month and our home equity slowly evaporate, I realize at least one of us might outlive our assets. My counselor warns me not to "catastrophize" this mentally and elicit unnecessary anxiety. My worst case scenarios may never materialize.

I'm working on it and often turn to prayer, humor, and yes, gratitude, for all the tender mercies that have come our way from coping with this devastating disease—one day and another loss at a time.

17

Long-distance Caregiving

MARIAN SHEEHAN

My knowledge of long-distance caregiving comes from two experiences. First, I took care of my mother who lived in another state and had Alzheimer's disease. Now, since her passing four years ago, I have been the facilitator for Alzheimer's Association long-distance caregivers support group in Seattle. I continue to learn so much as I listen to the stories and ideas that group members share each month.

Long-distance caregiving is not necessarily harder or easier than being close by. It's just different with a unique set of challenges. When you are far away from the person you are trying to care for, you go for long periods of time relying on other peoples' reports or trying to glean information over the phone. When you do go visit, it can be an intense, overwhelming, and exhausting few days with impossibly long to-do lists.

One advantage of a being long-distance caregiver and visiting the person for a few days is that you may get a much better sense of the person's true functioning, especially if you are able to stay under the same roof with him or her. I most often flew down from Seattle to my mom in California for three-day weekends. My mother was able to keep on her toes for the first day of my visits.

On the second day, some of her memory lapses were apparent. By the third day, she was exhausted from keeping on her toes for two days, and her deficits became very apparent. As hard as it was to see her at her worst, it was very helpful in planning her care. My brother who lived close by our mom would visit for an hour or two but didn't have the opportunity to see the problems I was observing.

My mother was a petite woman but a bundle of energy. She was always fiercely independent, well organized, and a force to be reckoned with if she didn't like what you were doing. There was not a shy bone in her body. She loved and lived for her work as a speech-language pathologist and couldn't imagine ever retiring. "What would I do? I've got to keep working." Her mantra was "Never give up, just keep trying," which buoyed the spirits of her patients who stuttered or who had had disabling strokes.

After my father's death in 1983, Mom lived alone in the Southern California house she and my father had purchased in 1954. My brother lived just a few minutes away from Mom, my sister in upstate New York, and I in Seattle.

My mother's father developed Alzheimer's in his seventies; it was one of my mother's worst fears that she would too. Even though my mother had been repeating herself for years, she functioned seemingly well both at home and work. Yet my siblings and I became concerned about our mother's driving.

We had many discussions about what to do. Mom would simply not discuss her old age, her driving, or give us information about her finances, insurance, or even where she kept important documents. Sometimes when my sister or I was visiting Mom, we would rummage through her desk while she was at the grocery store or the beauty parlor, definitely a stealth operation. Our mother's physician was of little help, always saying Mom was "fine." We felt worried and powerless. Mom seemed unstoppable.

What allowed us to intervene was an email a concerned friend in California sent me. The friend had run into Mom at an event and was worried that she seemed confused. My siblings and I seized this opportunity. We arranged an afternoon when my brother would take the email to Mom to let her read it while my sister and I were on conference call. Much to our relief, it worked. My mother was mortified, but she did agree to see a neurologist and a neuropsychologist and let my sister come for a couple of weeks and get a handle on the bills, finances, and legal documents.

The following month, my sister spent two hectic weeks at Mom's organizing her financial records, closed down all but two credit cards (there were well over a dozen), set up automatic payments for recurring bills, and found the information she would need to handle Mom's bills online. My sister discovered that my mother was being swindled by a so-called financial-planner.

Mom was also pledging small donations to every organization that contacted her, legitimate or not. My sister created an invaluable document, "Everything You Ever Want to Know about Mom," which listed contact information for doctors, hairdresser, plumber, utilities, bank and credit card accounts, insurance policies, and more. My copy quickly became dog-eared.

I had scheduled an appointment with my mother's geriatrician so my sister could meet the doctor. Beforehand I had written the doctor a letter with our concerns. In particular, I asked for help in getting Mom to stop driving. The doctor either did not read my letter or did not take it seriously. After the ten-minute office visit, the doctor's parting words to my mother were, "You're doing great. Keep driving. Keep working. Keep traveling."

The neurologist was much more helpful. He required that Mom have a neuropsychological assessment before her neurology appointment. The neuropsychologist felt that Mom was still functioning in the average range for eighty-seven-year-olds but diagnosed Mom with mild cognitive impairment. That diagnosis was a testament to my mom's strong pre-onset cognitive skills and her masterful covering-up. The neurologist referred Mom for an occupational therapy driving assessment, which she failed. She began taking some medications. I have often wondered if Mom might have functioned better or more happily had we gotten her started on medications earlier.

My sister interviewed homecare agencies that we might use in the future. For forty years, my mother had repeatedly stated, "I will not live with any of you kids, and I will not go to a nursing home." Mom did have the foresight to have purchased long-term care insurance and had the assets to afford a live-in caregiver. We wanted to honor her wishes.

Getting Mom to accept help was a different matter. We hired someone to assist with bill paying. The second time the gentleman came, Mom refused to let him in, insisting she didn't need any help. That was discouraging, but at least now we had a handle on Mom's affairs and a home-care agency we could call when the time came.

That time arrived two months later when Mom fell in a parking lot and fractured her pelvis. Typical of my independent, never-give-up mom, she drove herself home with a fractured pelvis. The hairline fracture wasn't diagnosed until an MRI two weeks later, but Mom was in enough pain that she agreed to a caregiver three mornings a week until her condition improved.

When I called one morning a few days later, Mom was alone, terrified, and in a state of panic because she couldn't get out of bed. That incident frightened Mom enough that she herself called the caregiver later that day and asked her to spend the night. Mom was never alone again.

We were fortunate to be able to keep Mom in her beloved home until she passed away three and a half years later. It was a very difficult three and half years. I flew down for a three-day weekend every four to six weeks during that period. I called her almost every day. I dashed to answer my phone every time it rang anticipating yet another problem or crisis.

My sister and I have had the what-could-we-have-done-differently conversation several times, but neither of us has ever been able to come up with anything specific that would have made it any easier. Alzheimer's is an unavoidably hard journey. In hindsight, we should have gotten my mom on hospice sooner, but we made the best decision we could at the time.

I have vowed to my children that I will *try* to be more cooperative if I develop what seems to be a familial Alzheimer's disease. I have made my wishes about care very clear. I have purchased long-term care insurance. I have signed a driving agreement my kids can show to me should they become concerned about my driving. I am working on writing a letter to my future self, reminding myself how important being cooperative is for everyone's well-being, mine as well as others'. While I'm not sure this letter will convince the future me, it is an attempt to grow old gracefully.

There is much I wish I had realized when I started on the journey of caring for my mother. These are my lessons from the School of Hard Knocks, offered because I learned them late and with difficulty:

Contact the Alzheimer's Association and learn about the wealth of resources offered. I tried a couple of different support groups before I found the long-distance caregivers group. My first night in the group I left thinking, "I so belong in this group." The group became my lifeline, and I always felt better after a meeting. I wish I had started going sooner.

Embrace the idea of therapeutic fibbing. This can be hard for caregivers who are uncomfortable being less than completely honest, but the benefits are tremendous. Reminding someone that her husband or mother is dead elicits feelings of shock and grief at the "news" every time it's repeated. What is the harm if someone thinks it is 1972 or that she's going to the prom next week? To correct such inaccuracies serves no purpose and may frighten, anger, or agitate the person.

Communication is paramount when trying to take care of someone long distance. Establish lines of communication with the person (as appropriate), with other family members, with paid caregivers, and with doctors. Email has made communicating much easier. Copying emails to family members who are not taking an active role in caregiving will at least keep them in the information loop. Ask doctors if they will email.

Be as concise as possible when communicating concerns to doctors. Doctors are more likely to read a half page of bullet points than a three-page narrative and more likely to take your phone calls if you are brief and to the point.

Try to find some watchful eyes when a parent is still at home without help. Talk to a neighbor or friend of your parent's, exchange contact information, and let the person know you would really appreciate a phone call if he or she notices anything awry. Once when I was visiting Mom, I intercepted the mail carrier who handed me the mail but insisted on talking with Mom. He said, "I need to see her and speak with her every day." Unbeknownst to us, he had been checking on Mom for two years.

Plan your visits with a list of what you hope to accomplish. Track down phone numbers and set up appointments before you go. But don't forget to spend enjoyable time with your loved one. Much on to-do lists can wait for the next visit.

Know that family squabbles are the norm. When people call interested in the long-distance caregivers group, they will often sheepishly say, "My sister and I can't agree" or "My brother thinks there's no problem," and apologize for their "weird" or "dysfunctional" family.

Some family members may never take an active role in caregiving. Standard advice is that families should commit to cooperation and share the burden. In reality, often one or two family members bear most of the weight, despite requests to others for participation or help. To keep expecting that someone will or should get involved or to continue feeling resentful that they won't only adds stress. Try to accept that life is unfair and go on doing the best you can.

Give yourself permission to grieve from time to time. When you're a long-distance caregiver and unable to visit frequently, the person's decline between visits can be shocking and upsetting. Your sense of loss can hit hard once you return home.

Taking action by volunteering may help combat feelings of helplessness. Sign up for the annual Walk to End Alzheimer's. Join a community or church program to visit homebound seniors. One woman in my group said she feels helpless about her father's decline, but by volunteering to participate in an Alzheimer's research study, she is helping to find a cure for this terrible disease. Wouldn't that be wonderful?

18

Not a Punch Line

KEVAN ATTEBERRY

My family moved to Washington State when I was almost six years old. Other than during college, I've lived my whole life within five or six miles of my childhood home. I still see people I went to school with—some from the first and second grade—and consider myself lucky to have such deep roots.

I was interested in art from the day I could hold a crayon and have been lucky to carve out a career that embraces that. I've been a graphic designer and illustrator and animator working for myself for years and currently am focusing my energy on a true love of mine, illustrating children's books. But my biggest claim to fame, so far, is in creating Clippy, the Microsoft Office paperclip.

Even though we went to the same high school, I didn't meet Teri till about seven or eight years after graduation. She was a year older, an athlete, and frighteningly pretty. I was ill-dressed, awkward-looking, and hung out with a crowd that was well removed from athletics. I knew who she was, but our paths never crossed.

So meeting her at the age of twenty-five moonlight bowling with friends seemed serendipitous. Of course we found out ten years later from those same friends that it was a set-up. It worked. Two years after that evening moonlight bowling, we married. We had two sons, and life was grand.

Teri initially worked in a couple of law offices and then went on to work in the offices of a mainframe computer company. After several years there and looking for a change, she took a sales position with a company that sold advertising specialties. And eventually she went out on her own. She liked the freedom of sales and meeting and working with people. She developed a good clientele of repeat customers and did well for years.

At some point, she started making mistakes. Nothing big at first, but eventually it started costing her clients—and us money. She'd get orders wrong; we'd have to eat the cost. She began losing clients until her business was down to just about nothing. I was watching this all unfold with some concern and took the opportunity to discuss what I thought was her inattention but to no avail. She became defensive, and I let her sort it out.

At the same time her business began suffering, she began forgetting little things in our day-to-day lives. I would get irritated or annoyed at her asking me or telling me the same thing over and over. Most of the time when I would remind her what we were doing this evening or that she just saw her sister on Tuesday, she would say, "Oh, yeah," and remember that she already knew that. Eventually when I would remind her of something I had told her multiple times, it would be as if she was hearing it for the first time.

But she would not let her memory be a topic of discussion. She'd get angry if I brought it up and tell me it was just a part of menopause and it would pass. It didn't; it kept getting worse. Friends and family began pulling me aside asking me about Teri. Wondering if she was all right. Wondering about her propensity for repeating things and asking the same questions over and over. I'd tell them that I was concerned too, but she was not willing, in fact adamantly opposed to, talking to a doctor about it, insisting, as things got worse, that it would pass.

Because her job as a sales rep for advertising specialties was, for all practical purposes, through, she took a succession of jobs that relied on her well-experienced administrative and office skills. Each of the jobs was short-lived due to her inability to comprehend the requirements and tasks of the job. Even clearly spelled-out and printed instructions didn't help.

She was getting discouraged and, I could tell, a little concerned, but she would still not let her memory be discussed. I knew it was more than her memory; it was the ability to execute simple tasks that she could always do before—the remote control for the television, the microwave, which knob was for which burner on the stove. And simple tasks became more difficult, like trying to follow recipes and signing onto the computer and checking her email.

Her final job was working for her brother who owns a manufacturer's rep company. He had hired her, knowing she was looking for work, to handle simple administrative things. He called me after a couple of weeks and told me it just wasn't working out. She could not do the simplest computer tasks, even with the steps printed out in front of her; she had gotten lost going to deliver something to a customer; filing confused her, etc.

He wanted her to see the doctor, too, so he told her, as her brother and as her boss, if she did not make an appointment to see someone about this he was going to fire her that day. She reluctantly agreed, and we began the testing. He kept her employed and on his insurance through the testing.

When she got the diagnosis, we were stunned. We worried about things like a tumor or brain cancer or even strokes. But we had never heard of younger-onset Alzheimer's disease and certainly didn't plan on it. Up to that point, Alzheimer's was, to me, hardly more than a stupid punch line of any number of jokes made at the expense of someone forgetting something. But my best friend's dad had been suffering from it for years. Three months after Teri's diagnosis, he would die from it.

We decided from the very beginning that her disease was something that we would have to share. We had a large caring group of friends and family, and they would all want to know. I felt a need to evangelize about it. Because I had never heard of younger-onset Alzheimer's, I wanted to make sure others were aware of it. It became apparent when we began telling friends and family about it that I was not the only uninformed person. Most everyone was as shocked about Teri having it as the fact there even was such a thing.

Once we got the diagnosis, Teri's brother let her go, and we moved her over to my insurance. We also had to switch medical networks and were lucky enough to wind up at the Memory Disorders Clinic and Dementia Health Services at the University of Washington School of Medicine.

We joined a group of other younger-onset patients and caregivers there for a monthly appointment. They were wonderful there and got us started down this path in several ways, including hooking us up with the Alzheimer's Association's regional office where we joined separate support groups—a caregivers one for me, a patients one for Teri. And recently, they started a support group for adult children of parents with younger-onset Alzheimer's, which both our sons, who are in their twenties, attend.

As Teri's disease has progressed, I've had to make adjustments. There are many more things that are my responsibility now. I moved my studio that I had in Pioneer Square for the past eight-plus years home. Working at home has been a challenge, but I'm starting to feel more comfortable with it now. I've worked mostly for myself the past thirty years and continue to do so.

I've taken jobs along the way, but they were all short term or contract. Now I don't believe I'll be able to take any kind of job that won't let me work remotely. As each month passes, it becomes more and more apparent that I need to be here much more often for Teri. So really, I'm lucky that I work for myself from home for now. The challenge is just keeping the work coming in.

Teri is not at that stage where I can't leave her for a few hours by herself. I know the day will come when that's no longer something I can do. I use the ability to leave the house for a few hours to take care of errands, meet friends, or hole up in a coffee shop to write. Working in the creative field, I have to avoid interruptions. Home has a lot of interruptions. I'm figuring tricks out as we go.

I still feel like an evangelist about this. I want everyone to understand what Alzheimer's is and how prevalent it is. It's a heartless disease, and I know that as I get older others around me will develop it. It's inevitable. With knowledge, maybe research will be better funded. Maybe solutions will be found.

So, I volunteer my services whenever the Alzheimer's Association asks me, whether it is to speak at a function or design a wine label for a fundraiser. I've participated in their walk to raise funds the past two Septembers, also claiming the title of the largest individual fundraiser both years. And Team Teri Atteberry will be walking again this fall.

I still get angry sometimes. I still get sad. And once in a while, I'll step back and look at this all from a distance, and it seems so surreal. How did this happen to me? To Teri? To us? What about all the things we wanted to do? Places we wanted to go? It all seems terribly unfair. But, we keep coming back to our mantra—it is what it is; let's make the best of it.

Part Four

Self-care and Renewal

*For memory is a blessing: it creates bonds
rather than destroys them.*

– Elie Wiesel

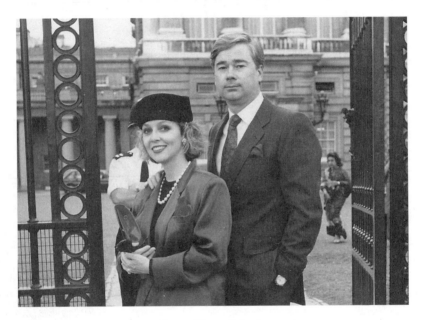

Jan and Barry Petersen

19

Lessons Learned

BARRY PETERSEN

Jan was diagnosed with younger-onset Alzheimer's disease in 2005. She was fifty-five. The diagnosis was done by a neurologist with considerable experience and knowledge of the disease.

Her diagnosis turned me into a caregiver. Unlike her doctor, I had no experience or knowledge to handle this new job. Most of us don't.

A family caregiver is chosen not by training but by geography. You are the nearest person to the person with the disease. She or he is a wife, a husband, a mother, a father, or a sibling. You love this person and take on the responsibility for caregiving.

Here are seven lessons that I learned the hard way.

Lesson One: You will never get ahead of this changing disease. You watch and respond to what the person is doing and go to bed thinking you have it under control, and the next day (or ten days later), there will be new and often aberrant behavior.

In Jan's case, she developed a phase I called the "Anger Monster" that hit about one to two in the afternoon, lasted for several hours, made her outraged at everything and pretty much everyone around her, and then faded as if on a train timetable promptly at four o'clock when she shifted into making-dinner mode. And suddenly she was happy.

Other people with Alzheimer's disease will, for instance, wake up and demand the morning paper and breakfast at 2 a.m. explaining that they "need to get ready for work" when, in fact, they retired years ago. One day they can cook a lovely dinner, and the next they turn the burner to high heat and blissfully walk away for a nap. One day they know their way around the house; the next and without warning, they walk outside and get lost.

On this issue, family caregivers can be divided into two groups. The first understands that nothing is predictable and realizes how this leads to exhaustion from battling a disease that keeps changing the rules. The second group would be those who think they have the situation under control, and this group can be generally referred to as delusional. In time, pretty much all of us will end up in group one.

Lesson Two: The disease will shrink your life. As the person you care for needs more, you have less of a life outside of caregiving. Friends fade away because you don't have time for them. Exercise, dining out, hobbies—all these things are at risk of ending. The danger is that most of us don't notice. It happens slowly, gradually, and because you are becoming more consumed caring for the person you cherish.

Caregivers run the risk (the statistics tell us) of dying before the person with the disease because the emotional and physical burdens escalate. Those who have come through this look back and see how much it took from them. If you are starting this journey, then make a promise: you will take care of YOU. As a wise person warned me in the midst of this, I could not care for Jan if I were dead. Surprisingly, that was not obvious to me until someone pointed it out to me. That is how deeply a caregiver gets drawn in and how much a caregiver can lose perspective.

Lesson Three: Call a lawyer. Immediately. Very few people have wills or trusts set up to accommodate the changes caused by this disease. With this diagnosis, there is a sudden and urgent need for powers of attorney for financial and health care decisions. Insurance beneficiaries may need to be changed. Trusts may need to be retooled. The person with the diagnosis may still be competent enough to sign papers. Neither you nor anyone else can know how long that will last. And if the cost of redoing wills and trusts seems burdensome, then wait and see how much more it is going to cost getting this done when your loved one cannot sign papers. It's the difference between buying a basic Ford or shelling out for a Cadillac.

You are on your own in this. The person you are caring for cannot help and may soon become difficult and uncooperative on money and legal matters. If that person is a husband or wife who handled the family finances (as Jan did in our lives), that phase is over. Either you get this part right, or you get it wrong. And there are plenty of consequences for getting it wrong. I got it wrong. What would have cost a few hundred dollars for the correct powers of attorney at the outset of this process took thousands of dollars in legal fees to correct a few years later.

And money set aside for other purposes may now be needed for caregiving. Brace yourself for a financial meltdown. Here is a heartbreaking example. A man told me how much time and money he spent caring for his mother at home and then after he moved her into assisted living. He spent what it took. But, he asked, what words do I use to tell my teenage daughter that I have now used all the money we set aside for her college education?

There are remarkably few insurance benefits that cover costs associated with Alzheimer's, unless you bought a specific long-term care policy. If you think Medicare will cover years of assisted living (as opposed to nursing home care), you are wrong as of this writing. At prices hovering in the range of six thousand dollars a month for assisted living, family funds can evaporate rapidly. That's seventy-two thousand dollars a year and then the year after, and on it goes.

Lesson Four: Realize when it is time for assisted living. From talking with others in this situation, I can say this with certainty... almost no one gets this one right.

The caregiver puts it off for financial reasons, but more often, the people I've met delay it because they believe they have an obligation to keep the person at home and cared for by the family. Emotions are dulled by exhaustion, guilt, and sometimes depression from the demands of being a caregiver. That can degrade the ability to make this critical decision. The default mode for most people is: I can struggle through this for a week/month/year longer. In my case, I had a live-in caregiver at that point. She suggested it was time to start looking into assisted living. Why at that particular time, I asked. That is the next lesson.

Lesson Five: Protect yourself. Unfortunately, most of us do this badly. When my caregiver sat me down on a lovely, sunny afternoon and said the words "assisted living," my first response was that Jan had changed but certainly not that much.

Jan has changed, she said, but that was not the real point. She looked at me and said rather bluntly, "You are going down." She was a trained nurse who monitored my escalating blood pressure and overall health, and she was scared at what she was seeing in me.

Sometimes, this decision has to be made based on what you, the caregiver, are experiencing and not the person with the disease. When, not if, it reaches the point that it is overwhelming for you, the caregiver, you waited too long. That is not a criticism but a bellwether, a way to know when you are now past the time you need to act.

Lesson Six: Caregivers are people until they stop being people. They can so easily lose themselves in caring for someone else. But as the process goes along, the one with Alzheimer's knows the caregiver less. You give ever more time, effort, and resources, and the person you are caring for appreciates this less. It is not personal and not a reflection on how or what you are doing. This disease, by its nature, is taking your loved one away along with awareness and memories. That means the demands on you increase, but the appreciation from the person can disappear.

Lesson Seven: This is the toughest lesson. You, the caregiver, have a life that can and must extend beyond Alzheimer's. If you let the demands of caregiving take you down, you will have failed. If you let the demands of caregiving ruin your health, you will have failed. If you let it rob the future that will come after caregiving, you will have failed.

Sounds harsh, but it is the truth. You can sacrifice everything to this disease—time, money, friends—but you are a fool if you also sacrifice yourself.

It is easy to lose perspective in the midst of being an Alzheimer's caregiver, so let me share some thoughts from being on the journey. There is life after this. The hope is (but it is not certain, depending on what this disease takes out of you) that you will outlive the person for whom you are caring.

In my case, I was caregiver to a wife I loved. We shared careers and experiences living and working in San Francisco, Tokyo, Moscow, London, and Beijing. I am a correspondent for CBS News, and Jan also worked across the world for CBS News, CNN, ABC News, and others. The disease took all this away from her and her away from me. And it layered stress onto my life that was already about unpredictable travel and sometimes life-threatening danger in very bad places where people kill people and journalists can get in the way.

Somewhere along my caregiver's journey came the realization that almost everything about my life had changed, and along the way, so had I. I never believed that I would be killed (no journalist does), but now it seemed even more important to stay alive so I could care for her.

We think Jan's Alzheimer's started in the early 1990s in small ways until it grew to the point of recognition in about 2000 (as we thought back on how she was then) and then to the formal diagnosis in 2005. I placed her in assisted living in 2008. But I had lost her as a wife and lover years before.

I was healthy (for this I give thanks) and suddenly looking at something called the rest of my life without Jan. Odd as it sounds, until I placed Jan into a facility, it never occurred to me to think about the rest of my life. I stood there, at the doorway of the facility where I was leaving her behind, and slowly realized that everything we had created and all that we had been was over. I vaguely recall that it was a sunny day in the Seattle area. I clearly remember how that day ended with me weeping on a hotel room floor in a fetal position.

But that could not be the end. Alzheimer's took Jan. It could not take me as well.

In time I reached out, met Mary Nell who found me (and my job) tolerable, and in late 2009, I left Asia to be with her in Denver. I consider myself lucky because I found that rest of my life. That same year, we moved Jan to an assisted living facility in Denver where we can watch over her.

Of all the things that being an Alzheimer's caregiver demands, this may be the hardest to accept and the most important to learn: you and your life must continue. No one can tell you the how of doing this, but I can suggest to you the why. I believe that this disease is like a person, something to be hated, something that wants not just the person we love and care for but also stalks every caregiver as well. It wants us. It wants two people.

Someday there may be a cure. There may even be a vaccine to prevent Alzheimer's. But for now it is, as doctors put it, 100-percent fatal. So going on, having a life after caregiving is how we beat Alzheimer's. Tough lesson. Learn it, and it will save your life.

20

God and Alzheimer's

SUSAN RAVA[1]

On a beautiful July morning, I looked from our cottage porch down to Lake Michigan where I saw my eighty-one-year-old father-in-law, Paul, swimming alone straight out into the lake toward Milwaukee some sixty miles away. Paul was a fine swimmer and a determined man. He and my mother-in-law, Silvia, had emigrated from Italy because of the racial laws against Jews at the beginning of World War II. True, Paul had begun to lose his keys and confuse names. But my husband, John, and I shrugged off what we considered typical old age.

That morning, I ran down to the beach, yelled, and waved. Paul didn't hear me because he had taken off his hearing aids. An inner compass must have told him to turn around. When he came ashore, I said, "Paul, we have a no solo swimming rule. Please don't swim alone." Polite as ever, he agreed. But after lunch, I glanced at the lake and once again saw Paul swimming alone toward Milwaukee. A year or so later, Paul was afloat in his own inner world. Doctors tested him and

---

[1] "God and Alzheimer's" is adapted from an article that was published in the *Huffington Post*, October 3, 2013, Religion section and is reprinted with permission.

then diagnosed him with probable Alzheimer's disease. That summer of Paul's solo swims was the last time we invited him to vacation with us in Pentwater, Michigan.

That Paul's Alzheimer's disease might cause a spiritual crisis seldom entered my day-to-day thinking. I did mention to my pastor—I am a lifelong, mainstream Presbyterian—that we were having a hard time with our aging parents, an understated, Calvinist approach. Stubborn, I was intent on forging my own path as parent to our parents without allowing care-giving to dominate our lives. I did begin to mutter "Help me" prayers on Sundays.

These first cries of anguish came as our four parents, one after another, developed Alzheimer's disease over a four-teen year period. Their disease began to create invasive, unpredictable, and unmanageable crises, which strained John and me individually and as a couple. Alzheimer's was proving chaotic with its unexpected twists and turns: Paul's temper tantrum in his bank, my father's hidden silver, my mother-in-law's cries of *aiuto*, Italian for help. Caregiver fatigue set in. God seemed of little comfort.

Paul, the first of the four parents to pass away, died at age eighty-five. By then, John and I were so tired that we blocked out signs of Alzheimer's disease developing in his mother, Silvia. One summer, she came to Sunday lunch soiled and confused. She forgot a date with me for a political gathering. A friend reported that Silvia could no longer manage renewing her theater tickets. Both John and I denied or ignored these signals and did not let ourselves imagine that his mother was a victim of Alzheimer's herself. Yet as we slowly faced the reality of his mother's illness and my own father's Alzheimer's, my prayers grew more intense.

The next round of prayers—and I was fast running out of confidence that anyone was listening—became a "How can this be?" and "Please, someone somewhere, help me in the midst of this unpredictable situation." When Silvia and my father's disease overlapped, caregiving began to overwhelm me. Disorder invaded our lives every time a charge nurse or a well-meaning friend telephoned to report bad news. I was desolate when we authorized alarms on Silvia's bed and wheel-chair. Alarms and dulling medications flew counter to the precepts of my Judeo-Christian heritage: do unto others; honor thy mother and thy father; be ye kind one to another.

I became numb and worn out. John grew numb, worn out, and ill. We didn't stop taking care of our parents long enough to recalibrate our lives, much less to analyze faith issues. Yet my own deep-seated faith and John's spiritual imperative to take care of one's own drove us. So we continued, begrudgingly keeping the commandment to honor our parents.

We often questioned why we continued to carry on. Montana became our secret escape code when either of us was at wit's end. Once on the way to a nursing home, I told myself that I could bail out, keep on driving, and flee to Montana. Defiantly, I wondered what commanded me to stay, to field charge nurse calls, or to sit at arm's length from my mother-in-law so she wouldn't pinch me. The free and wide skies of Montana tempted me.

Nonetheless, a voice in the center of my being told me that I belonged not in Montana but with my parents. What voice was this I heard? For me, it was God who directed me to accompany my father and mother in their decline.

Nor did John choose Montana. He carried on, unswerving and loyal, nourished by his own inner source. His parents had brought him out from World War II European fascism and provided a full American life. By their own enduring ties with Italian family, they exemplified a spiritual imperative, born of the Judeo-Christian background we share. It says to care for one another within the family, no matter the circumstances.

Yet the God of that caregiving period was not a caring presence. I could no longer summon up the Supreme Being I had long believed in, a supreme being who had provided me with a vision of possible order and goodness in the world. How would such a being allow old people to lose their minds, allow a disease to ravage the core of their characters? Prayer became a moan or a sigh.

In my fatigue and despair, I came to the point of wishing the mothers dead. I asked myself if it was sinful to wish my loved ones dead and wondered how far I had strayed from that biblical imperative to honor my parents. Everything in my life was upside down: my husband no longer an anchor; my sweet mother-in-law cranky and prone to biting and pinching; my organized mother unable to execute the plans she loved to make. God did not figure in this mess.

After ten years of caring for one parent after another and of despairing consultations with John, social workers, and my Thursday-morning walking friend, I felt utterly weighed down by responsibility. If God had abandoned those with Alzheimer's disease, I was certain God had also forsaken me. At last, I recognized my need for professional, spiritual help. I was, after a decade of caregiving, full of self-pity and far removed from an imperative to honor my parents. I went to see my pastor and lay myself bare.

I hoped Daniel, my pastor, would know whether the pieces of this fragmented, doleful period of my life composed a pattern, a coherent story if viewed differently. Daniel would discern, perhaps, what God had in store for me. In my heart, during the days of Alzheimer's dying, I wondered where God was, why deaths piled one on top of the other. I began, "So I came today to see what all this caregiving means. And my role. Basically, why me?"[2]

---

[2] Susan Rava, *Swimming Solo: A Daughter's Memoir of Her Parents, His Parents, and Alzheimer's Disease*, Sewanee: Plateau Books, 2011, 239-240.

We sat quietly for a moment. I hoped Daniel was interceding for me with God. "Susan," Daniel said, "God says to Moses before he approaches the burning bush, 'Take off your sandals because you are standing on holy ground.' You and John are walking on holy ground as you make this journey of dying with your parents. Holy ground, life and death. I hope you know that."[3]

In that moment, I needed counsel and comfort. I didn't grasp the profound nature of God's words to Moses and how this seemingly abstract verse applied to me. Naïvely, I wished my pastor, like a magician, could strengthen and reassure me that our decisions were the best John and I could do, that I wasn't falling apart, and that God wasn't judging how anguished, how conflicted, and how tired we felt. Somebody needed to lift the guilt that haunted me: not paying enough attention or paying too much attention; not spending enough time or spending too much time; making yet another imperfect decision; feeling furious at myself, my family, and my parents for this ending to their lives. I longed for my pastor to wipe away that awful sense of never caregiving quite right.

Yet with hindsight, I see that God took my hand and steadied me. God indeed led me onto hallowed ground. In occasional flashing moments, our parents showed the essence we had known and reminded us of their lives well lived. On my mother's ninety-fifth birthday just months before her death, she cooed and rocked her newest great-grandson, baby Emmett. Such moments strengthened John and me, individually and as a couple. The memories of hard times fade. Our sense of having been true both to our beloved parents and to ourselves survives.

I had counted on someone, maybe Daniel, to answer my question about God's place in this dread disease that afflicts both patient and caregiver, albeit in different ways. While in

[3] *Ibid*, 241.

the moment, I was disappointed, I now know that no solace exists for a caregiver, no panacea for difficulties faced. I have still not heard adequate words of counsel or comfort for either an Alzheimer's patient or a caregiver. "I am so very sorry," is the only response I can imagine to one on an Alzheimer's journey.

After my crisis of faith, God has resurged like a phoenix. We and our family honor all four parents each July on that very beach in Michigan where Paul first set out to swim solo. We are not alone. We rejoice that together we trod this holy ground.

21

Mastering Our Dread of Alzheimer's

ANTHONY D. ROBINSON[1]

You've heard it. Maybe you've said, "If that happens to me, just shoot me!" "That" is dementia or Alzheimer's disease.

Others mutter, in some ways more darkly, about saving up meds for an overdose. What are we saying and why?

I spend part of the summer caring for my ninety-three-year-old mother at a family cabin in Oregon. She has moderate dementia. She loves to be at the cabin, though shortly afterward, she doesn't remember that she's been there. This summer I also read several books on dementia. And I pondered the eight years that my dad had Alzheimer's before his death.

All of this leads me to think we ought to think twice about the "just shoot me," and other off-hand comments and lame attempts at humor.

Not to say the prospect of dementia isn't scary. It is. We are scared. According to a 2010 Metlife study, people over fifty-five dread getting Alzheimer's more than any other disease.

---

[1] "Mastering Our Dread of Alzheimer's" was first published in *Crosscut* (September 22, 2011) and is reprinted with permission.

And, as Margaret Morganroth Gillette pointed out in a recent *New York Times* Op-Ed ("Our Irrational Fear of Forgetting"), "Greater public awareness of Alzheimer's, far from reducing the ignorance and stigma around the disease, has increased it."

But there's a kind of self-fulfilling prophecy at work here. Dreading isolation, we isolate. Dreading a diminished life, we diminish. Dreading the loss of our powers, we disempower.

All the books I read on dementia agreed. Half of us who live to be eighty-five will experience some form of dementia or cognitive impairment. (They also note that dementia is a symptom not a cause. About 60 percent of the time, the cause of cognitive impairment is Alzheimer's. But 40 percent of the time, dementia is caused by other things like a stroke, Parkinson's or Huntington's disease, or one of a host of other causes.)

So if in a group of ten friends all live to be eighty-five, half of you will likely have some form or level of cognitive impairment. We should shoot everyone? Probably not.

Susan and John McFadden in their fine book, *Aging Together: Dementia, Friendship, and Flourishing Communities*, argue that dementia needs to be viewed as a disability.[2] As we have learned to include and accommodate people with other disabilities, we need to do so with those who experience dementia.

They tell a story of when Al, a larger-than-life extrovert with a bawdy sense of humor, missed several weeks of Rotary, and rumors began to circulate. Finally, Al appeared at a meeting. When time came for announcements, Al approached the podium. "Some of you have probably heard that I have Alzheimer's disease," he told the hushed room. "Well I do. For a while I was too embarrassed to come to meetings.

---

[2] Susan and John McFadden, *Aging Together: Dementia, Friendship, and Flourishing Communities* (Baltimore, MD: Johns Hopkins University Press, 2011).

"But a friend said to me that if Rotary could put up with me the way I was before I had Alzheimer's, they can put up with me now. I may mess some things up. I may not remember your name. But if I can deal with Alzheimer's, you bastards can too." Al received a lengthy round of applause. In the coming weeks, Al's dementia became simply a part of who he was rather than something to speak of in whispers. He was able to attend Rotary for two more years before his condition worsened.

Yes, dementia and Alzheimer's are tough. But they aren't the end of life. There's still a person there. There's still someone who can experience joy. Someone who can grow and contribute to the growth of others.

Ours is a "hypercognitive" society where rational function is highly valued. Part of what my experience with my own parents and others with dementia has taught me, confirmed by my reading, is that people with dementia operate more on emotion than on cognition. They feel stuff. They are in touch with their feelings. They read and respond to the emotional state of those around them. It's not how we operate, by and large, but is that such a bad thing?

This does means that relating to people with dementia requires adapting. Trying to make them adjust to our version of reality is often counterproductive. Quizzing them, for example, about what day it is or what they had for breakfast, only stirs anxiety. I like the joke about George W. Bush visiting a care facility and asking an elderly woman, "Do you know who I am?" She answers, "No, but if you go to the front desk, they can tell you!"

Laura Wayman, in her very helpful book, *A Loving Approach to Dementia Care*, notes, "You will never win an argument with someone with dementia."[3] So don't try. Wayman teaches the "affirmative response" method.

---

[3] Laura Wayman, *A Loving Approach to Dementia Care* (Baltimore, MD: Johns Hopkins University Press, 2011).

As we prepared to leave the family cabin at summer's end, my mother began to obsess about my grandmother's collection of ceramic roosters and chickens, which sits on the shelf above the stove. She insisted that we always took them all down and put them away before we left, which had actually never happened. Arguing the point was pointless. So I simply said, "Right, OK, don't worry. I'll do that after you leave and before I close up the cabin." The chickens came up two or three more times. I said the same thing. It was OK.

One day this summer, I took my mother and another older friend on a cookout by what we call Hurricane Creek in the Wallowa Mountains. As I built a fire for hot-dogs and s'mores, my mother sat at the picnic table. I noticed she was swinging her legs like a ten-year-old. She was in her "joy zone." She loves the mountains and trees, the sky and clouds. As the fire caught, she said (repeatedly), "Isn't that a nice fire!" The next day she had no memory of our cookout, but she had been fully present, legs swinging with the music of the stream and enjoying it at the time. It occurred to me that she was doing what the Buddhists urge on us all: living in the moment.

Better than muttering "just shoot me" will be coming to grips with our fears, learning from those who experience dementia, and becoming more inclusive of people who, as Al put it, may mess up and may not remember your name. There are worse things. Like those of us who don't have dementia forgetting their names and forgetting them.

22

Bread for the Journey

RITA BRESNAHAN[1]

What was curious to me, at the onset of Mom's disease, was that I, too, felt disoriented. Although I had read volumes on Alzheimer's, I could find no clear road map, no specific time frame to mark the passages. Yes, research literature does describe stages and sequences, but it offers no clear definitions. What's more, I find each stage and sequence to be quite subjective, as each person is so different in unique and unpredictable ways.

In my disoriented stage, I began pondering—which is almost a way of life for me. Ever since I was a teenager, I have been an avid student of any subject that sheds light on how we create meaning throughout this life of ours. How are we to respond to life's deep questions, such as "Who am I?" "Why am I here?" "Where am I going?" "How do I get there?" "Where am I now?" Through the years, I have pored over hundreds

---

[1] "Bread for the Journey" is excerpted from Rita Bresnahan, *Walking One Another Home: Moments of Grace and Possibility in the Midst of Alzheimer's* (Ligouri, Missouri: Liguori/Triumph, 2003) and is reprinted with permission.

of books on psychology, religion, philosophy, mythology, and ritual, all of which have left impressions on my soul.

It is only natural, then, at this soul-searching time, that I should insist on asking myself, *So, if there is no clear road map out there, Rita, how will you find your way as companion through the Alzheimer's journey?* It is only natural that I should reflect on which rich insights and familiar treasured sources might provide a sketchy map for me, might guide me, might offer me fresh perspective and meaning. The words of Spanish poet Antonio Machado's were both unsettling and reassuring: "Traveler, there is no path. Paths are made by walking."

I found inspiration from many sources, but one book by Phil Cousineau, *The Art of Pilgrimage*, spoke to me most deeply. His wise words: "We can transform any journey into pilgrimage with a commitment to finding something personally sacred along the road," resonated with how my own journey was unfolding.[2] Only as I opened to the sacredness of this image did I begin to understand the uniqueness and the depth of such a pilgrimage through Alzheimer's. My writing soon began to bring together these two unlikely companions—Alzheimer's and spirituality—through the metaphor of a pilgrimage.

Pilgrims leave their comfortable everyday surroundings to venture, at least for a while, into challenging and unfamiliar territory. Often they journey to places where a holy presence is felt, places credited with healing powers.

Consistently, I felt a holy presence when I was with my mother, and her tiny nursing-home room offered healing at many levels. True, absurd dilemmas often arose, stirring strange and unwelcome feelings in me. At such times, I would become impatient or preoccupied or even depressed as I witnessed Mom's downward spiral. Watching someone I

---

[2] Phil Cousineau, *The Art of Pilgrimage: A Seeker's Guide to Making Travel Sacred* (San Francisco: Conari Press, 1998).

love so much fade before my very eyes was not easy and often made me feel helpless. What could I do? Being helpless seemed pretty much a given in this situation. I myself needed help—help from a power beyond my own, help tempering my testy and challenging times.

But this much remained clear, however. I could do nothing about Mom's deteriorating condition. What I could do something about was my own behavior, my attitude toward what we were facing. I could bring into our interactions greater love and compassion, more patience and flexibility. In each given moment, this is my call ...

Yes, we walked one another home faithfully, Mom and I, in our pilgrimage through Alzheimer's. In tender and sacred times ... through the darkness and the light ... step by step. Through each story. Each encounter. Through each day. Each moment.

> *Life is so full of meaning and purpose,*
> *so full of beauty—*
> *beneath its covering ...*
>
> *Courage, then, to claim it ...*
> *and the knowledge that we are pilgrims together,*
> *wending our way*
> *through unknown country, home.*
>
> – *Fra Giovanni*

Pilgrims frequently speak with great fondness and even awe of teachers they meet along the way, those who open up their minds and their hearts, helping them face what lies ahead. In this pilgrimage with Mom, I often find myself wondering, *Could it be that in her Alzheimer's, Mom is teaching me something profound, even something of the essence of life?*

Not always have I been open to the possibility that Mom had wisdom to share with me—certainly not as an adolescent, nor even as a young adult. That both Mom and I are such strong-willed, stubborn women often got in the way of our relationship. Over the last twenty-five years or so, however, that has markedly changed. Especially now, it has become crystal clear to me that my mother is indeed my teacher. And my decision to receive her teaching with an open heart makes all the difference to me in this journey: I am able to *listen* to Mom from a deeper place. I then listen to *myself* there too—and to God's voice as well. It feels like throwing open a window to let in the fresh air of awareness. I am grateful.

When I was a young girl and someone gave me a gift, Mom always prompted, "What do you say?" From her, I first learned to say "Thank you." Even more, she taught me how to live in a grateful spirit, to appreciate the little things as well as the big. So, I am left with these questions: what can help me remember to carry that piece of wisdom with me, to count whatever blessings are still mine? Here Mom is in a nursing home, enduring countless losses, yet her attitude is nearly always a positive one. In fact, "thank you" are the words I hear her speak most frequently.

And she is constantly surprised—by flowers that have been in her room for days, or by visitors who just step out of the room for a while. "Oh," she exclaims, smiling broadly at their return, delighted to see them as if they have just come. She lives David Steindl-Rast's words: "An inch of surprise can lead to miles of gratefulness."

I intend to welcome into my life more of this surprise-gratefulness combo. Also I will continue to challenge myself: how can I shift the spotlight of my awareness away from regret, away from what I can no longer do, from what I no longer have—and then very deliberately focus that spotlight on the many gifts of life I do continue to enjoy?

Mom's abiding gratefulness and playfulness and her gift of staying in the present speak powerfully of what truly matters. These practices offer bread for the journey that are nourishing to both of us. Again and again, Mom teaches me directly by her own actions these special qualities of a pilgrim spirit. I pray for the grace in my own life to match her faithfulness.

> *This old woman ...*
> *isn't my mother,*
> *is not what I think.*
>
> *She's a spiritual master*
> *trying to teach me*
> *how to carry my soul lightly*
> *how to make each step*
> *an important journey,*
> *every motion and breath*
> *anywhere*
> *as though anywhere*
> *were the center*
> *of the earth.*[3]

---

[3] Poem by Betsy Sholl in Tillie Olsen and Estelle Jussim, eds., *Mothers and Daughters: An Exploration in Photographs* (Reading, PA: Aperture Press, 1987), 245.

23

The Bird That Sings in the Night
OLIVIA AMES HOBLITZELLE

When faced with one of life's greatest challenges—living with Alzheimer's disease—how do we continue to live with some measure of acceptance, equanimity, and a peaceful heart? When my husband received that tentative diagnosis at age seventy, this question became urgent, especially for me, his caregiver throughout his six-year illness until his death. Yet we were fortunate; we were both psychologists as well as steeped for many years in Buddhist meditation and the wisdom traditions. These fields all deal with the nature of the mind, emotions, and spirit. This gave both of us a lot of resources for handling his illness.

Time is the great healer. Since it's over ten years since my husband's death, I now have the gift of perspective. I can look back with more objectivity to what really helped—the insights and discoveries that I want to share here. My hope is that they will provide some useful approaches to caregiving, whatever your circumstances.

My overarching assumption, then and now, was that the spiritual dimensions of caregiving would help to lighten the burdens of that role. That will be unique for each of us; it depends on our spiritual orientation, or the absence of it. In either case, we need to make sense of life, even how to find meaning in suffering. Because I'm an optimist by nature, I knew that there had to be some gifts, even grace, in the midst of this difficult illness.

The first insight may come as a surprise. It occurred to me during an ordinary moment of preparing dinner one night while Hob, as my husband was called, sat waiting passively in the family room as I worked at the stove. I experienced a shift of perspective, a sudden moment of illumination. At the soul level, I thought to myself, we'd made a deal to go through this together. Hard as it was, there was no mistake. The question was how we would live through his illness as consciously and lovingly as possible.

These became two key words for me: consciously and lovingly. Mostly, this perspective was far in the background, but I sometimes remembered it in crisis moments and felt grateful for what I called the "meta" level of our situation. Whether the phrases "soul level" or "meta level" resonate with you or not, it's another way of looking at how we share certain experiences with the people in our lives. Call it our shared destiny. As with any new perspective, this idea of the soul level of our journey helped me accept the challenges of caregiving.

"What do you call this disease I have?" asked Hob one day. "Is it called horse blinders?" When I chuckled and explained that the word was "Alzheimer's," he, the former English professor, broke into laughter and said, "That's not bad for the wrong word! 'Horse blinders' both scans and rhymes with Alzheimer's."

Hob was blessed to have a great sense of humor and often approached his illness with that playfulness. That may be somewhat unusual because many people don't know that they have some form of dementia or choose not to talk about it. The main point is that whenever we can find the lightness or humor in a situation, it lightens the burden for everyone. The energy of the moment shifts. Something softens and loosens up. As serious as any illness is, it is still possible to find some lightness. For me, that became something to affirm and cultivate. It certainly made our lives easier.

When I first learned that we were now living with Alzheimer's disease, I knew I needed help. I went to talk with a longtime friend, an *anamcara*, or spiritual friend, as the Celtics call it, though in this case it was a Buddhist teacher named Tulku Thondup. Of all the places where I sought help, I found his guidance the most inspiring. His main message was to invite me to see my caregiving role as part of my spiritual practice. It doesn't matter if you have a different spiritual orientation or none at all because what he said contained universal truths far beyond any particular tradition.

His first statement stunned me, yet it ultimately became the most inspiring. He said, "This illness is difficult, but take it as a training, a teaching, and a blessing." I could appreciate what he meant with the first two words, but a blessing? He must be misinformed, I thought to myself, but over time, amazingly, even though Hob's illness would lead to death, I came to see the blessings along the way. Life became simpler, slower, with more time to appreciate the little things. His situation blew my heart open with compassion. His vulnerability invited new tenderness between us. The kindness of friends and family supported us. On the other hand, to be realistic, I also fell apart. I raged (to myself, not at him). I wondered if I could make it through. I grieved. Yet in spite of all the harsh, heartbreaking realities, the love between us deepened, and there were moments of grace, of blessings. That was what my teacher friend meant.

T.T., as he's known, went on to say that I could cultivate what are called the perfections in the Buddhist tradition. Perfection is a tricky word, but this is more about intention, something we aspire to. The perfections are the positive qualities common to all traditions: generosity, patience, loving kindness, equanimity (meditation), effort, and wisdom. Cultivating these qualities becomes part of one's spiritual practice, if that is one's perspective about living with mindfulness and compassion in difficult circumstances.

"Think about it," he said. "The simple act of giving someone a spoonful of food involves these qualities—patience, generosity, steadiness, compassion."

He had used the most humble example to illustrate this teaching. Of course I forgot it! But I also remembered it from time to time, for he had framed caregiving as spiritual practice. To give two examples, when I felt frustration burning through me (call up patience!), when I felt exhausted (call up effort and equanimity!), when I thought I couldn't stand the pressure, I'd remember compassion. What was it like for *him* to have his mind disappearing? Walk in another's shoes, as the saying goes, and feelings of compassion arise. In truth, T.T.'s vision was anchored in practicality. Cultivating positive qualities—the perfections—was one way to approach something as difficult as caring for someone with dementia. That was his gift to me as well as for many with whom I've shared his story.

Anyone who has cared for someone with dementia knows well the emotional challenges of this illness, the whole range of emotions, including worry, frustration, boredom, grief, anger, desperation, fear, heartbreak, and so on. I sometimes needed help from family and friends to acknowledge how hard it was, lean on them, ask for help, and find my own ways of handling the intensity. Sometimes the combination of exhaustion and frustration broke through my coping mechanisms; I just needed to cry, ventilate my feelings to someone, or find an outlet for my anger. I'd get in the car, drive off, and roar until the blocked feelings erupted into tears. They were tears of release and relief. I wasn't angry at Hob; I was angry at the situation. Also I was determined to keep my emotional intensity to myself as I saw how increasingly sensitive he had become and how easily my irritation or impatience upset him. Our sadness, however, we sometimes shared.

This also led to a simple practice that helped me to cope. When I felt emotionally strained in some way, I'd sometimes remember to stop whatever I was doing, put my hand on my heart center, and repeat silently to myself, "May I have compassion for myself. May I have compassion for myself." I would focus on the softness and openness of the heart to soften around some powerful emotion. I'd coordinate the words with my breath so that I was breathing in compassion and breathing out the difficult emotion. I'd feel the warmth rising in the heart center. I'd feel some shift in my energy, however subtle. Sometimes I'd extend that wish or prayer to him or even to everyone—"all beings" as the prayer says—who was struggling with caregiving for someone with dementia. Mostly, however, I just needed to help myself in that moment!

Many years before Hob's diagnosis, we'd been very close to a friend who was living with cancer. At one of our meetings, she shared a message sent to her by a friend that she had found very inspiring. I was only in my early forties at the time, but when I heard this message, I copied it from the letter. I immediately recognized its value for sometime in the future and started a file entitled "Wisdom and Aging." This first entry came from Teilhard de Chardin, the French philosopher, theologian, and mystic, as he wrote about his experience of growing older.

> In my younger years, I thanked God for my expanding, growing life; but now, in my later years, when I find my physical powers growing less, I thank God also for what I call the grace of diminishment.

The grace of diminishment. Some might hear this phrase and react, "Who wants diminishment?" It's a tough challenge, to be sure, but it's the reality of growing older. That we live in a youth-oriented culture that wants to deny the aging process is no help; aging, death, and dying are in "the natural order of things." That is another phrase that I find comforting. That phrase, too, helps with acceptance; it invites us to live with the reality of life, hard as it may sometimes be. With further reflection on de Chardin's words, we may recognize that grace may break through, in spite of the losses and grief.

Life slows down and gives time to appreciate the little moments that get lost in overly busy lives, to draw together around someone who is ill—with the kindness, generosity, and love that may grace the most difficult situations. Granted, it is an exalted view of aging but that is why it is inspiring. On several occasions, I reminded Hob of those words. For both of us, this phrase was also embedded with the courageous way in which our friend had lived through cancer. That too is a reminder that how we live through something difficult can become an inspiration for others.

I've left to the end the most valuable of all the approaches that came into our journey with Alzheimer's and specifically my role as a caregiver. Hob and I had both had almost thirty years of meditation training and practice. Granted, this is far from being the natural way for many people, but any form of meditative activity that involves working with the mind will be helpful. That includes other disciplines like tai ch'i chuan, ch'i kung, tae kwan do, and so on, or even some forms of repetitive exercise. The key is training the mind. We need to understand the power of awareness.

We need to familiarize ourselves with the vast range of mental and emotional states that contribute either to our happiness or to our suffering. Through the long and gradual process of learning to stop, sit still, and be with whatever arises, this process—both simple and profound—cultivates acceptance, equanimity, kindness, and compassion. Our resistance to various circumstances in our lives is the cause of much of our suffering. We judge. We want things to be different. We may not even realize that we're in a quiet (or not so quiet!) struggle with our life. Meditation invites us to step out of that struggle and gradually develop the capacity to be with and accept the vastness of human experience, the whole range from joy to sorrow.

I'm not sure I could have gotten through the endless changes of caregiving without the reliable companion of meditation practice. One practices bringing mindfulness, or moment-to-moment awareness, to daily life. That helps immeasurably how we respond to all the demands of caring for someone with dementia. Our calm and steady presence may be one of the greatest gifts we can offer to our loved one. For ourselves, a meditation practice helps us to live more consistently in the present moment and, in particular, not get entangled with the worries and fears about the future that often accompany living with any serious illness.

As for Hob, I had to remind him to meditate, which we usually did together. I once asked him how it was now that his mind was in new realms. He answered, "It's a lot easier now because there aren't so many thoughts!" We had a good laugh over that one, a reminder of how much humor helps to lift the burdens of loss.

I'm sure most of us who have served as caregivers have had those understandable moments of anxiety, self-doubt, and judgment—the range of afflictive emotions—that make us wonder whether we're going to get through. Here, another element comes in: faith. Faith may come from our spiritual tradition; it may be something we naturally feel; it may arise from our meditation where a deep conviction emerges that, at some level, all is well no matter what is happening. This sure sense is beautifully expressed by Rabindranath Tagore's poetic words that I read long ago:

> Faith is the bird that feels the light and sings when the dawn is still dark.

Acknowledgments

This anthology is the result of the collaboration of many colleagues and friends over the course of several years. First, my thanks to Bob Le Roy for writing his gracious foreword to this book. Second, to Patricia Hunter, Washington State Long-Term Care Ombudsman, my thanks for her encouragement from the project's inception. Third, my gratitude to Linda Whiteside, Keri Pollock, and Joanne Maher at the Western and Central Washington State Chapter of the Alzheimer's Association for their unstinting support with all aspects of this project. Finally, special thanks to Julie Scandora and Susan Rava for their fine editorial assistance and Sheryn Hara for her enthusiastic embrace of this project.

I owe a profound debt of gratitude to the writers in this anthology for sharing their stories. Their dedication inspired me. Thanks, too, to Alexandra Kovats, Robert and Peggy Wallace, John Townsend, Kevin Peterson, Thomas Broughton, James Chuck, Al and Joyce Ferkovich, Elizabeth Gray, Hugh Huntley, Fred Kronacher, Robert Johnson, Barbara Petura, Joann Byrd, Gerri Haynes, Lisa Mayfield, Larry Johnson, Roger

Roffman, Sara Robertson, Deborah Swets, Diane Douglas, Lynn Samford, Joel Van Etta, Peter Jabin, Candace Dempsey, Merrillann Hutchinson, Sharie Todd, and especially my late Washington State University colleagues, Sally Savage and Bill London, for their encouragement.

I would be greatly remiss if I did not express a belated word of gratitude to my late theology and ethics professor, Robert McAfee Brown at the Pacific School of Religion at Berkeley who taught me about the power of sacred stories. Bob's courageous example has shaped my own life in ways too numerous to enumerate. To Troy Duster, Ched Myers, Cynthia Moe-Lobeda, Sharon Moe, Mary Petrina Boyd, Steve Thomason, Julie Braybrooks, Eldon Ernst, and Mary Rose Bumpus, my appreciation for their wisdom and friendship.

Finally, to my family and wider community of friends, my grateful thanks for their love and support.

Selected Bibliography on Alzheimer's Caregiving

Barbas, Nan, Laura Rice-Oeschger, and Cassie Starback. *The Shapes of Memory Loss: Stories, Poems and Essays from the University of Michigan Medical School and Health System.* Ann Arbor: University of Michigan Library, 2013.

Basting, Anne Davis. *Forget Memory: Creating Better Lives for People with Dementia.* Baltimore, MD: Johns Hopkins University Press, 2009.

Bayley, John. *Elegy for Iris.* New York: Picador, 1999.

Block, Stefan Merrill. *The Story of Forgetting.* New York: Random House, 2008.

Boss, Pauline. *Ambiguous Loss: Learning to Live with Unresolved Grief.* Cambridge, MA: Harvard University Press, 2000.

———. *Family Stress Management: A Contextual Approach.* Thousand Oaks, CA: Sage Publications, 2001.

————. *Loving Someone Who Has Dementia: How to Find Hope while Coping with Stress and Grief.* San Francisco, CA: Jossey-Bass, 2011.

Bresnahan, Rita. *Walking One Another Home: Moments of Grace and Possibility in the Midst of Alzheimer's.* Liguori, MO: Liguori/Triumph, 2003.

Broyles, J. Frank. *Coach Broyles Playbook for Alzheimer's Caregivers: A Practical Tips Guide.* Fayetteville, AK: J. Frank Broyles, 2006.

Chittister, Joan D. *Scarred by Struggle, Transformed by Hope.* Grand Rapids, MI: William B. Eerdman's Publishing Company, 2005.

Coste, Joanne Koening. *Learning to Speak Alzheimer's: A Groundbreaking Approach for Everyone Dealing with the Disease.* Boston, MA: Houghton Mifflin Harcourt, 2003.

Cousineau, Phil. *The Art of Pilgrimage: A Seeker's Guide to Making Travel Sacred.* San Francisco, CA: Conari Press, 1998.

Fazio, Sam. *The Enduring Self in People with Alzheimer's: Getting to the Heart of Individualized Care.* Baltimore, MD: Health Professions Press, 2008.

Feil, Naomi, and Vicki de Klerk-Rubin. *The Validation Breakthrough: Simple Techniques for Communicating with People with Alzheimer's and Other Dementias.* Baltimore, MD: Health Professions Press, 2002.

Genova, Lisa. *Still Alive.* New York: Pocket Books, 2009.

Gibbons, Leeza, James Huysman, and Rosemary DeAngelis Laird. *Take Your Oxygen First: Protecting Your Health and Happiness while Caring for a Loved One with Memory Loss.* Brooklyn, NY: LaChance Publishing LLC, 2009.

Gibson, John. *Family Matters Matter: Stories of Flexibility, Reconciliation, and Healing.* Charleston, SC: BookSurge Publishing, 2008.

Gibson, John, and Judy Pigott. *Personal Safety Nets: Getting Ready for Life's Inevitable Changes and Challenges.* Seattle, WA: Safety Nets Unlimited, Ltd., 2007.

Gruetzner, Howard. *Alzheimer's: A Caregiver's Guide and Sourcebook.*, New York: John Wiley & Sons, Inc., 2001.

Hedreen, Ann. *Her Beautiful Brain.* Berkeley, CA: She Writes Press, 2014.

Helfgott, Esther Altshul. *Dear Alzheimer's: A Caregiver's Diary & Poems.* Yakima, WA: Cave Moon Press, 2013.

Heston, Leonard L., and June A. White. *The Vanishing Mind: A Practical Guide to Alzheimer's Disease and Other Dementias.* New York: W. H. Freeman and Company, 1983.

Hoblitzelle, Olivia Ames. *Ten Thousand Joys and Ten Thousand Sorrows: A Couple's Journey through Alzheimer's.* New York: Jeremy P. Tarcher/Penguin, 2008.

Hughes, Holly, ed. *Beyond Forgetting: Poetry and Prose about Alzheimer's Disease.* Kent, OH: The Kent State University Press, 2009.

Innes, Anthea, ed. *Dementia Care Mapping: Applications across Cultures*. Baltimore, MD: Health Professions Press, 2002.

James, Oliver. *Contented Dementia: 24-Hour Wraparound Care for Lifelong Well-Being*. Manville, IL: Vermilion, 2009.

London, Judith L. *Connecting the Dots: Breakthroughs in Communications as Alzheimer's Advances*. Oakland, CA: New Harbinger Publications, 2009.

Lustbader, Wendy, and Nancy R. Hooyman. *Taking Care of Aging Family Members: A Practical Guide*. New York: The Free Press, 1994.

Mace, Nancy, and Peter Rabins. *The 36-Hour Day: A Family Guide to Caring for People Who Have Alzheimer's Disease, Related Dementias, and Memory Loss*. Baltimore, MD: Johns Hopkins University Press, 2011.

Magniant, Rebecca C. Perry. *Art Therapy for Older Adults: A Sourcebook*. Springfield, IL: Charles C. Thomas, Publisher, Ltd., 2004.

Martin Gary A., and Marwan N. Sabbagh, eds. *Palliative Care for Advanced Alzheimer's and Dementia: Guidelines and Standards for Evidence-Based Care*. New York: Springer Publishing Company, Inc., 2010.

McFadden, Susan, and John McFadden. *Aging Together: Dementia, Friendship, and Flourishing Communities*. Baltimore, MD: Johns Hopkins University Press, 2011.

Pearce, Nancy D. *Inside Alzheimer's: How to Hear and Honor Connections with a Person Who Has Dementia.* Taylors, SC: Forrason Press, 2007.

Petersen, Barry. *Jan's Story: Love Lost to the Long Goodbye of Alzheimer's.* Lake Forest, CA: Behler Publications, 2010.

Power, Allen. *Dementia beyond Drugs: Changing the Culture of Care.* Baltimore, MD: Health Professions Press, 2010.

Rava, Susan. *Swimming Solo: A Daughter's Memoir of Her Parents, His Parents, and Alzheimer's Disease.* Sewanee, TN: Plateau Books, 2011.

Reiswig, Gary. *The Thousand Mile Stare: One Family's Journey through the Struggle and Science of Alzheimer's.* Boston, MA: Nicholas Brealey Publishing, 2010.

Shenk, David. *The Forgetting—Alzheimer's: Portrait of an Epidemic.* New York: Anchor Books, 2003.

Sifton, Carol Bowlby. *Navigating the Alzheimer's Journey: A Compass for Caregiving.* Baltimore, MD: Health Professions Press, 2004.

Small, Gary. *The Memory Bible: An Innovative Strategy for Keeping Your Brain Young.* New York: Hyperion, 2002.

Small, Gary, and Gigi Vorgan, *The Alzheimer's Prevention Program: Keep Your Brain Healthy for the Rest of Your Life.* New York: Workman Publishing, 2011.

Snyder, Lisa. *Living Your Best with Early-Stage Alzheimer's: An Essential Guide.* North Branch, MN: Sunrise River Press,

2010.

Taylor, Richard. *Alzheimer's from the Inside Out*. Baltimore, MD: Health Professions Press, 2007.

Troxel, David, and Virginia Bell. *A Dignified Life: The Best Friends Approach to Alzheimer's Care, A Guide for Family Caregivers*. Deerfield Beach, FL: Health Communications, Inc., 2002.

Wayman, Laura. *A Loving Approach to Dementia Care*. Baltimore, MD: Johns Hopkins University Press, 2011.

Zeisel, John. *I'm Still Here: A New Philosophy of Alzheimer's Care*. New York: Penguin Group, 2009.

Contributors

KEVAN ATTEBERRY has illustrated a number of award-winning children's books, including *Tickle Monster, Frankie Stein*, and his latest, *Halloween Hustle*. He recently penned his own picture book, *Bunnies!*, which Harper Collins will publish in two volumes in January 2015. His biggest claim to fame is in creating Clippy, the paperclip helper in Microsoft Office. Kevan lives in Bellevue, Washington, with his wife, Teri.

VIRGINIA BENSON is a native of St. Louis and a graduate of Washington University. Her pre-caregiver work was raising her three now-adult children, a brief sojourn in graduate school, and later in public relations for nonprofit organizations. She is an avocational musician and hopes one day to resume activities that feed her intellectual curiosity.

RITA BRESNAHAN has been an educator and psychotherapist for over thirty years and has a PhD in psychology from the Union Institute in Cinncinati, Ohio, and Certificate of Study in Aging at the University of Washington's Geriatric Education

Center. Rita has worked extensively with issues of aging people and their caregivers and led more than one hundred workshops on "Aging as a Spiritual Journey" in a variety of settings. She is the author of *Walking One Another Home: Moments of Grace and Possibility in the Midst of Alzheimer's*.

BOB BROOKS is retired from the navy. Prior to that, he served in the US Army during the Vietnam War. After military service, he worked for the Boeing Company in Seattle and later for Panasonics Avionics Corporation. Since 2007, Bob has been a caregiver for his wife, Linda.

NANCY GOULD-HILLIARD is a retired journalist and media relations specialist with a thirty-year career in education reporting at community newspapers and university news operations at Washington State University and the University of Idaho. She recently helped update the Mercer Island History book and volunteers through Rotary, church, alumni groups, and PEO. Her work as a two-time census taker and genealogist for scores of families tags her as a "finder," thus extending her public information skills into the private domain. She has been caregiver for her husband, Bob, for nearly fourteen years of their thirty-two-year marriage.

ANN HEDREEN is a Seattle writer, producer, director, teacher, and voice of the KCBS radio commentary and blog, *Restless Nest*. She has won many Emmys and other awards, including a recent first place in science and health reporting from the Society of Professional Journalists. Her film, *Quick Brown Fox*, won a Nell Shipman Award for Best Documentary. She recently published a memoir, *Her Beautiful Brain*. Ann began her career at the City News Bureau of Chicago.

ESTHER ALTSHUL HELFGOTT, a Seattle nonfiction writer and poet, earned a PhD in history from the University of Washington. Her essays, "Witnessing Alzheimer's through Diary and Poem—Dear Alzheimer's: Why Did You Pick Our Sheltered Lives to Visit?" (2010) and "Diary of My Husband's Illness: After His Death—Still Witnessing Alzheimer's" (2012) appear in *The Journal of Poetry Therapy*. Her poems on Alzheimer's have been published in *Floating Bridge Review*, *Beyond Forgetting: Poetry and Prose about Alzheimer's Disease*, Holly Hughes, ed., and *Northwest Prime Time*. She is the author of *The Homeless One: A Poem in Many Voices* and *Dear Alzheimer's: A Caregiver's Diary & Poems*.

OLIVIA AMES HOBLITZELLE is a Boston-based writer, therapist, and teacher. She taught in the field of behavioral medicine where she pioneered in ways to bring meditation, yoga, and cognitive therapy into the medical domain to treat stress-related and chronic illness. She helped to develop one of the first training programs in mind/body medicine in the country and trained health professionals through Harvard Medical School. She is author of *Ten Thousand Joys and Ten Thousand Sorrows: A Couple's Journey through Alzheimer's*.

STEVE KNIPP works as the human resources director for St. Vincent de Paul in Seattle and has become increasingly specialized in the area of Alzheimer's caregiving as he supports his partner through living with the disease. When time allows, he enjoys camping, swimming, going to the movies, and hanging out at coffee houses with friends. He and his partner, David, live together with their chosen family, and Jetta, their ten-year-old miniature schnauzer.

PEGGY MITCHELL, a native of Springfield, Illinois, is the second of four daughters of Robert and Margaret Jackson. She did her undergraduate studies in sociology at Southern Illinois University at Edwardsville and holds a license as a practical nurse. She has been married to Marc Mitchell for twenty-one years and has two sons, Jabari and Kamali. She is the primary caregiver for her mother, who has lived with her family since 2007. She enjoys sewing and gardening as hobbies and is active in her church, as well two nonprofit disability organizations.

KATHLEEN O'CONNOR is the author of *The Alzheimer's Caregiver: Strategies for Support, The Buck Stops Nowhere: Why America's Health Care is All Dollars and No Sense,* and *Embracing Two Lives: A Journey of Love, Loss, and Healing.* A published poet, she also wrote a guest column for four years on health care policy and politics for the *Seattle Times.* Her articles and op-eds have appeared in publications such as the *Washington Post, Washington CEO, HMO Magazine,* and *Health Care Informatics.*

BARRY PETERSEN is an award-winning correspondent for CBS News where he has worked for the past three decades. He is now based at Denver, Colorado, where he reports for the *CBS Evening News* and *CBS Sunday Morning.* Until September 2009, he was based in both the CBS News Tokyo and Beijing Bureaus, commuting between and living in both cities. Petersen returned to Asia in 1985 after almost five years in the London Bureau (1991–95). Prior to that, he was CBS News' Moscow bureau chief and correspondent (1988–90). His first Tokyo posting was 1986–88. He joined CBS News in 1978 and worked at the Los Angeles and, later, San Francisco bureaus. Petersen's book, *Jan's Story: Love Lost to the Long Goodbye of Alzheimer's* was published in June 2010.

SUSAN RAVA is a writer and former senior lecturer in French literature at Washington University, where she earned her PhD.

She has published pieces in the *New York Times Book Review*, *Christian Science Monitor*, *Change*, and the *St. Louis Magazine*. Her short stories have appeared in the *Crescent Review* and *Prairie Schooner*. Susan lives in St. Louis, Missouri, with her husband. She and her extended family spend July on the shore of Lake Michigan where her memoir, *Swimming Solo*, begins and ends.

ANTHONY ROBINSON is the author of several books on theology and congregational life, including *Common Grace: How to Be a Person and Other Spiritual Matters*. He served four congregations in both rural and urban settings. In 2004, he completed fourteen years of ministry at Plymouth Congregational Church in Seattle. He contributed op-ed columns to the *Seattle Post-Intelligencer* and articles for magazines and journals, including the *Christian Century*. He is the president of a new program of leadership education and formation, the Congregational Leadership Northwest.

MARIAN SHEEHAN is a speech language pathologist and owner of a solo private practice in Seattle. She earned her PhD in speech pathology from the University of Minnesota and was an SLP for more than thirty years. Marian is the facilitator for the Alzheimer's Association long-distance caregivers support group and was a member of that group when her mother was alive. She is the mother of three children, two of whom were teenagers and the oldest in college when she was taking care of her mother in California.

STEPHANIE STAMM earned a PhD in religion and literature from the University of Chicago and now lives and works in southwest Michigan. A technical writer by day, she is also the author of a young adult urban-fantasy novel, *A Gift of Wings*, which is dedicated to her sister, Carol. Stamm is currently working on the sequel, *A Gift of Shadows*.

BABS TATALIAS is an artist. Whether she works with words or ink or people, her efforts are woven together skillfully and joyously. She also is a mother and teacher, who has been a mentor to scores of people in different ways in their professional and personal lives. She has worked in settings as varied as the corporate world, a Montessori school, and volunteer committees. Babs also enjoys her time spent in solitude in a yurt at her favorite retreat on Orcas Island, Washington.

STEFANIE TATALIAS divides her time between writing, yoga, being outdoors, and raising her children. She is the founder of Write Young Alaska and Anchorage regional advisor for the Society of Children's Book Writers and Illustrators. Her short stories have been published in anthologies, and excerpts from her novels have won awards. She practices and teaches yoga in Anchorage. Life's joys and sorrows inspire—and force—her to write every day.

CONNIE THOMPSON is news anchor and producer of consumer affairs segments for KOMO 4 News in Seattle, Washington. She is the recipient of numerous honors, including the 2006 Silver Circle Award from the National Association of Television Arts and Sciences. She also has been honored by Women in Communications, the National Transportation Safety Administration, Totem Council of Girl Scouts, and Big Brothers Big Sisters of Puget Sound, which established an annual award in her name for her more than two decades of support.

KARL THUNEMANN, a journalist for most of his professional career, was editorial page editor of the *Eastside Journal-*

American in Bellevue, Washington. A native Washingtonian, he graduated from the University of California, Berkeley. Karl also worked at the Western and Central Washington State Chapter of the Alzheimer's Association in Seattle.

JEANNE TRIPSANSKY is a cosmetologist and provides spa and wellness services at her salon, Spirals. In the two years since her mother's passing, she turned her attention to fitness training, earning educator certificates in Nia White Belt, Nia Green Belt, and Ageless Grace, which she currently teaches. Jeanne earned a Bachelor of Science degree in microbiology from the University of South Florida. She lives in northern Indiana with her husband, Richard, two rescued collies, and five stray cats.

ARLENE ZAREMBKA, an estate planning and elder law attorney, serves on the Public Policy Committee of the St. Louis Chapter of the Alzheimer's Association and the Legal Committee of the American Civil Liberties Union of Missouri. She has received numerous awards for work on behalf of civil rights and civil liberties. She lives with her spouse, Zuleyma Tang-Martinez, and their dog, Chispa.